# Focus on Professional Issues

First edition

Library of Congress Catalog Card Number: 75-27344
International Standard Book Number: 0-913654-14-0

Manufactured in the United States of America
by SCIENCE PRESS, Ephrata, Pennsylvania

# Nursing Digest
# Focus
# on Professional Issues

Edited by
the Editorial Staff

**Table of Contents**

# Attaining Control Over Professional Practice

## Ingeborg G. Mauksch

**Ingeborg G. Mauksch, R.N., Ph.D.** is professor and family nurse-practitioner, Department of Community Health and Medical Practice, School of Medicine, University of Missouri, Columbia.

Contemporary writers agree that an occupation's control over its practice is one of the essentials for gaining recognition. They contend that nursing, as an almost exclusively woman's group, has exercised only minimal control over the conditions of its practice in the past. Consequently, nurses have been relegated to a position of subservience and order-taking, or semi-professional status in the employment setting.

Condensed and reprinted with permission from *Nursing Forum*, Volume 10, Number 3, (September, 1971), pp. 232–238.

The prognosis for nursing's success in becoming an autonomous, self-directing occupation, according to these writers, varies from poor to somewhat hopeful. Because of their willingness to be subjected to the dictates of hospital administrators and physician employers, nurses have denied themselves the practice of nursing as a self-generated, autonomously guided service to people.

Will nurses continue to follow the route of the submissive employee who primarily carries out technical functions to implement physicians' orders? Or will nursing become an autonomous occupation, whose practitioners will be respected members of the health-care delivery team, participating equally as professionals in meeting society's demands for health- and illness-care?

The official approach nursing seems to have taken toward control over conditions of its practice is essentially expressed through the American Nurses' Association's Economic Security Program. However, the program, while manifestly directed at the control of economics, also includes the control of other conditions of practice which are of equal or greater significance to the profession and to society.

Attainment of control over professional practice can be attempted in many ways and in the pursuit of a variety of goals. In nursing, attaining control now seems to be directed toward obtaining better care for patients, thereby enhancing the nursing function. That the economics of nursing has been badly neglected is largely responsible for the current status of nursing practice. However, we must recognize that nursing's economic plight is not the sole substandard condition of relevance. Economics seems to have been selected as the main focus of nursing's strivings for control because it is the most tangible, readily describable, and socially understandable need at present. It may also have been recognized that as long as adverse economic conditions prevail, nursing as a career will not attract either the kinds or the numbers of entrants required to meet society's needs for health care.

Nurses are primarily employees. That their conditions of employment and much of their practice are dictated by employers who, for the most part, represent not-for-profit organizations contributes largely to the lack of control nurses are able to exercise. However, it would be simplistic and inaccurate to place all the blame on the shoulders of employers. In the past, nurses as a group have not attempted to exercise control and, in fact refused opportunities to do so. Furthermore, they have rarely participated meaningfully in decision making regarding the delivery of health care. Now there are signs that this may change.

Nursing has many questions to answer around the issue of control. Among the most significant: Is it possible for an occupation whose members are primarily employees to practice autonomously within the framework of an institutional employment setting? Can an occupation strive toward excellence in institutional practice without exerting the control necessary for that occupation to be sufficiently autonomous? Will tomorrow's nurses engage in autonomous practice within a variety of employment settings, assuming the responsibility to control their practice, and exhibiting accountability for quality of care delivered? Or, will they continue to remain the somewhat middle-level deliverers of services to patients, responding primarily to physician's prescriptions, and ultimately being replaced by other functionaries? Such crucial issues will require disposition in the not-too-distant future.

"Personal autonomy can be regarded as freedom to conduct tangential work activities in whatever manner one desires," states Engel. "Work-related autonomy for the professional, on the other hand, can be defined as freedom to practice in accordance with his training. It is this type of autonomy which appears to be critical for the individual professional if he is to provide the quality of service demanded of him by the profession and by the society." It is important, therefore, for an occupation to exercise control over conditions of its practice in order to be able to render the best services possible. Moreover, the manifest destiny of an occupation can be reached only if each member of the occupation is in control of his activities and attains the goals set forth by the group as a whole. Thus, it seems imperative that attempts at control attainment by isolated groups of nurses must gain the support of the whole profession. Only then can these strivings become institutionalized, thereby providing new norms.

If today's nurses are to support endeavors toward control attainment, they need to understand the nature and goals of assertive collective behavior. Otherwise, they will continue to reject it as a means to attain shared goals. Collective bargaining is by no means the only potentially successful form of collective behavior. The emphasis must be on the goals that collective behavior attempts to attain; that is, maintaining the core values of nursing and delivering high-quality nursing care under conditions conducive to such practice. By understanding why nursing is where it is today and why it has to work collectively to attain such goals, nurses may increasingly value their own practice, want to control it, and ultimately, assume accountability for its delivery.

# Toward a full profession of nursing: the challenge of the educator's role

*Marguerite J. Schaefer*

Nursing's task has been spelled out by the National Commission for the Study of Nursing and Nursing Education in the question: "How can we improve the delivery of health care to the American people?" Whether nursing ever becomes a full profession depends upon society's assessment of its performance with respect to this question. If nursing can make a commitment at a national level to an action program which it develops and implements, perhaps professional status will be forthcoming.

It is my thesis that those who deliver health care and who qualify by today's standards as professionals

**Marguerite J. Schaefer, D.Sc.** is professor of Administration at the University of Pittsburgh School of Nursing.

Condensed and reprinted with permission from the *Journal of Nursing Education*, Volume 11, Number 4, (November, 1972), pp. 39–45.

> **"If nursing can make a commitment at a national level to an action program which it develops and implements, perhaps professional status will be forthcoming."**

will retain that status only if they meet society's needs. Nursing will qualify as a profession only when it can and will do what is required of it. It is for this reason that we desperately need to establish national nursing goals wedded to society's needs. Michael Novak states in a recent article, "Politics as Drama," "No program becomes practical until its present base and future can be plotted out and interpreted to the society for whom it is cast."

Florence Nightingale wrote papers on sanitation, hospital administration, and health statistics as well as on nursing. She fought on many fronts because she ardently believed in the improvement of the care of the ill. She founded modern nursing and insisted on better education for nurses as essential components of an *array* of required reforms. During the past few years she would have learned about the extent of the health care problem, done her own analysis of the reasons for it, proposed new ways of delivering care and promoted them publicly and politically. The hour is late, but our credibility as concerned citizens, our status as professionals, and our needed contribution to health care can still be secured if we clearly state what we

believe future health care should be, how we think it can be delivered, and what responsibility we will assume for it. Nursing can act collectively as a Florence Nightingale if it but will!

This is not to suggest that nursing has no goals, or that nurses are unaware of the need for change. What is missing is a picture, national in scope, and a program of action. Highly polished descriptions of purpose have a hollow ring until they are translated into action. Individual nurses work hard to translate nursing's avowed purposes into action but individuals cannot do it alone. A national posture is required to cope with the mammoth task confronting us and to elicit the moral and financial support we need.

## THE EDUCATOR'S ROLE

Educators carry a heavy responsibility for the future of health care in this country. As is pointed out in *An Abstract for Action,* "When nursing meets the requirements for professional recognition on the counts of educational process and a unique body of knowledge, then it can be assumed that practice must and will follow." Educators at all levels of nursing education must assume that responsibility, and commit themselves to burying hatchets and making the compromises required for forward movement in an organized, cohesive manner. Particularly heavy responsibility lies with educators located in

**"The hour is late, but our credibility as concerned citizens, our status as professionals, and our needed contribution to health care can still be secured if we clearly state what we believe future health care should be, how we think it can be delivered, and what responsibility we will assume for it."**

universities, since it is there that one finds the concentration of personnel and resources needed to conduct research in nursing.

It is essential that educators take a leadership role in developing a position paper for national consideration. The recommendations of the National Commission document what is required for health care to advance through improved nursing practice. These recommendations could provide a base for planning and priority setting with the ultimate aim of designing a program of action.

Many other challenges face nursing. They reside in the analysis provided in *An Abstract for Action* of the reasons why nursing does not currently qualify as a profession. Strategies must be developed to achieve professional characteristics: high level of commitment, disciplined educational process, unique body of knowledge and skill, active and cohesive professional organization, and discretionary authority and judgment.

An attack on the problem of commitment has first priority because it is related to the acute need for increasing the size of nursing's leadership group. There is no possibility that nursing can become a full profession unless more nurses can be prepared for and persuaded to assume leadership roles.

Nursing has a leadership problem in part because it is predominantly a female occupation in a culture which has neither expected women to become leaders nor rewarded them for doing so. Many professional women have testified to the difficulties they face by virtue of their failure to fit the traditional female model.

Nursing is remiss in that, although it is the second largest women's occupational group, it has remained essentially uninvolved in the feminist movement. Nurse educators in particular, have enormous opportunities to help large numbers of students understand themselves better as women and to raise their level of consciousness. Nurses do not understand the significance of this movement for nursing leadership with respect to this and other problems faced by nursing in practice and in academe. These problems will only be solved at the grass roots level.

The recruitment of able women and men who will be leaders is increasingly in jeopardy because of nursing's failure to get involved in the women's movement. Nursing is seem by all who write about women's liberation as a field to which women

> "Nursing has a leadership problem in part because it is predominantly a female occupation in a culture which has neither expected women to become leaders nor rewarded them for doing so."

with limited aspirations are attracted. Donald McDonald, Executive Director of the Center for the Study of Democratic Institutions wrote:

> Women who are excited in the freshman year by the possibility of entering professional and research fields, by the time they are juniors, lower their aspirations to more "practical" fields (teaching, nursing, social work, secretarial-administrative work) which may be far below their abilities.

Recruiting men into the profession is important, but I hope the reason is because men have significant contributions to make to health care. To recruit men to help nursing meet the professional mark with respect to level of commitment and to provide leadership in the field is not only a colossal cop-out but a disservice to all women in this country. It should be remembered that the liberation of women in our society contains many elements of liberation of men as well. Do we have any idea how many men might opt for nursing careers if our culture viewed its work as something other than feminine?

Further, there is a connection between women's liberation and a national commitment by nursing to reform health care. It boggles the mind to think what nursing could do for women and for society if it would link social reform in health care to the feminist movement. Might not such a move attract more students with high leadership potential into nursing? Would we retain, to a higher degree, those active minds who become disenchanted with the passivity which dominates the nursing scene?

Before leaving the subject of commitment, I must mention that personal commitment to a profession or even to being the best possible practitioner of that profession is no longer sufficient. Professionalism in any service field does not exist in a vacuum but rather as part of a system. In the case of nursing, professionalism is tied to the health care system. Today's system is under heavy attack, and no matter how much we wish to deny it, nursing is also under attack.

The present health care system will change as a result of political action. Whether the changes under debate in Congress will provide better health care and whether revisions in the health care system help nursing maximize its contributions should be a matter of grave concern to all nurses.

> Politics is the art of creating actions by entire communities. Politics is the art of shaping many disparate social elements into social, not pri-

7

vate action. It is the art of directing societies. It includes the craft of acquiring and using power, and the craft of reconciling interests. But these are the instrumental crafts, subordinate to the overarching craft of directing societies from one state of being to another. [1].

When will faculties in schools of nursing recognize the need to become politically involved, to work with their students for reform in health care and to educate them in the "art of creating action?"

I have dwelt on the professional characteristic of commitment rather than speak to the other four professional characteristics (disciplined educational process, unique body of knowledge and skill, active and cohesive professional organization, and discretionary authority and judgment). This is because I believe that if nurse educators would concentrate on reforming health care and improving the condition of women, and would encourage nurses to become political animals, the rest would follow.

Women will not (in large numbers) participate in a disciplined educational process in a culture which paints a different ideal. Unless many nurses undertake a disciplined educational process, the research needed to establish a unique body of knowledge and skill is a dream. Discretionary authority and judgment will be won politi-

cally — locally within hospitals, at the state level with the passage of new nurse practice acts, and nationally with action programs which directly influence federal legislation. An active and cohesive professional organization might become a reality if the organization stood for reforms in health care which most nurses know to be necessary and could support, and if it fought for the liberation of women generally and for nurses specifically.

The challenge that nurse educators face, if nursing is to emerge as a full profession, is threefold. First, they should exert leadership in setting future directions for nursing, with improved care as the focus. Secondly, they must work to enunciate a national program of action and plan for its implementation. Lastly, the crisis in leadership must be faced as nursing's foremost internal problem. Short- and long-range goals for increasing the size of the leadership group are essential and should receive the highest national priority. The future of nursing and health care is to a large degree dependent upon meeting these challenges.

### REFERENCE

[1] Michael Novak, "Politics as Drama." *The Center Magazine,* a publication of the Center for the Study of Democratic Institutions, 5(3):9, 1972.

*Medicine marches on.*
*The law and ethics straggle behind.*
*We have the knowledge to prolong life.*
*Here, a Catholic theologian asks*
*if we have the wisdom to end it.*

# DEATH BY CHANCE, DEATH BY CHOICE

## *Daniel C. Maguire*

**Daniel C. Maguire** is associate professor of theology at Marquette University, Milwaukee, Wisconsin.

Condensed and reprinted with permission from the book *Death By Choice.* Copyright © 1974 by Daniel C. Maguire. Published by Doubleday & Company, Inc. An unabridged version of this article also appeared in *Atlantic Monthly,* (January, 1974) pp. 57–65.

About two million people die each year in the United States, and the American culture has finally decided to take note of this fact. Death in our day is having its belated due. It is slipping out from under denials and disguises and bursting into explicit, obsessive, and, at times, pornographic recognition. The overall meaning of this revolutionary shift in death-consciousness is probably one of gain and health and not of decadence and morbidity. Only in a mature culture can death be received and accepted as a natural companion of life.

Whatever the long-term cultural significance of our current concern with death, however, there are shorter-term questions which are now urgently addressing the moral consciences of mortal men. Basically, they arise from the fact that man is the only animal who may have death by chance or death by choice. He may also, in a reflective way, allocate death for others when he judges that certain values outweigh the need or right of others to remain alive. But it is no gentle irony that humans have traditionally been much quicker to justify the killing of others than the killing of self.

At any rate the problem of willful death-dealing has taken on new urgency because of revolutionary developments in medical science, the laggardly state of the law, and important shifts in moral outlook.

> ". . . humans have traditionally
> been much quicker to justify
> the killing of others
> than the killing of self."

Science, which once basked in the illusion that it was somehow "value-free," is suddenly up to its neck in value-loaded questions. Medicine becomes more and more involved with problems of ethics as it is repeatedly forced to ask itself if it *may* do what it suddenly and often surprisingly *can* do.

And, speaking of the surprising, medicine, which has been making all these quantum leaps in our century, suddenly finds itself bereft of an agreed-upon definition of death. The current terms "brain death" and "heart death" suggest an unsettling distinction, especially since you can have one without the other. The inability to define death, and the ability to create situations where death would appear to be preferable, are parts of the perplexing yield of scientific medical progress.

Are not the pressures for shaping a moral position on death by choice mounting with every medical advance? Could we not also expect that as infant mortality goes down and disease is further vanquished and population pressures on the earth's resources increase, there will be special challenges to the right to life of defective children? Note the words of Millard S. Everett in his book *Ideals of Life:*

My personal feeling — and I don't ask anyone to agree with me — is that eventually, when public opinion is prepared for it, no child shall be admitted into the society of the living who would be certain to suffer any social handicap — for example, any physical or mental defect that would prevent marriage or would make others tolerate his company only from a sense of mercy. . . . Life in early infancy is very close to nonexistence, and admitting a child into our society is almost like admitting one from potential to actual existence, and viewed in this way only normal life should be accepted.

Thus, what to some is unthinkable has been thought and written. Medical power with every victory over disease creates conditions that stir up moral questions about death by choice.

---

*". . . can the will of God regarding a person's death be manifested only through disease or the collapse of sick or wounded organs, or could it also be discovered through the sensitive appreciations and reasonings of moral men?"*

---

Medicine cannot distinguish between good death and bad death. As medicine has developed, it is geared to promoting life under all circumstances. Death is the natural enemy of the healing science.

Death, however, can at times be a welcome deliverance from a situation that has ceased to be bearable. Pneumonia has been referred to as "an old man's friend," since it often served, in days of simpler science, to shorten the old man's final agony. Actually, it was death that was the friend; pneumonia merely gave access to it. Now, of course, pneumonia usually can be contained and the old man lingers on in agony.

Dr. Eliot Slater, editor-in-chief of

the *British Journal of Psychiatry,* puts it in blunt language: "Death performs for us the inestimable office of clearing up a mess too big to mend; if we are going to intervene, then we must have at least some hope of doing this ourselves." What Dr. Slater is unambiguously saying is: If diseases such as pneumonia can be friends, why can we not be? Is it not within man's inherent moral freedom to recognize instances when death would be a blessing and to bring it about in ways that would be even more merciful than a bout of pneumonia? Must mortal man await the good pleasure of biochemical and organic factors and allow these to determine the time and the manner of his demise? Putting it in religious language, can the will of God regarding a person's death be manifested only through disease or the collapse of sick or wounded organs, or could it also be discovered through the sensitive appreciations and reasonings of moral men?

There is, of course, a big difference between not treating pneumonia, and overdosing a patient to accelerate the death process. Though omission and commission are different realities with a potential for radically different moral meanings, they have a suggestive similarity in that in both cases, someone is dead who would have been alive if a different decision (to act or not act) had been made.

Some of the most difficult cases in

point which medical progress has thrown at us involve children. At Johns Hopkins University Hospital, the parents of a mongoloid baby requiring surgery for survival refused to give permission. This case is not, by any means, unique but it received national attention in 1971. It took the baby fifteen days to succumb, during which time the hospital staff had to watch the infant struggle unsuccessfully for life. Many moral and legal questions were raised by this one incident. Should the parents have been made to take the child home and bear the pain of standing the death watch that their decision inaugurated? Should the state have taken legal charge of the baby away from the parents and then authorized the operation, or should a court order have overruled the parents' decision? If it was thought that the child's death would indeed have been a mercy, could it not have been accelerated by increasingly large doses of morphine? In other words, should a certain amount of commission be added to the fundamental omission of the operation?

Though the death of this child *may* have been a mercy, the dying was not. In fact, is this not a case where the omission might have been immoral without the act of overdosing to shorten the final fifteen days of torture? In other words, maybe omission was harder to justify in this case than commission. Or is the entire question of opting for this baby's death morally repugnant?

Dr. Warren Reich, a senior research associate at the Kennedy Center for Bioethics at Georgetown University, posed a hypothetical case at the meeting of the International Congress of Learned Societies in the Field of Religion in September, 1972. The case involved a girl who was born with spina bifida with meningomyelocele of the lumbar spine. The child lacked reflex activity in both legs and could not control her anal or urinary sphincters.

Hydrocephalus develops in 90 percent of these cases. Even with a shunt, the child would have a fifty-fifty chance of being mentally retarded. Bowel control would be a lifelong problem for her. Kidney failure is a constant danger and the most common cause of death for children with this affliction.

In the panel discussion of this case, Dr. Harmon Smith of Duke University Divinity School noted that until ten years ago, about 80 percent of such babies died and that today 75 percent survive. Thus, again, medical advance brings on troubling new moral questions. Should this baby have been allowed to die from the meningitis that would normally ensue in such cases? Or should the doctors have begun at once what would be for the child a lifetime of extraordinary care? The panel considered only these two options.

In the discussion, it was suggested that there were other options, such as the direct termination of life. This was an option that no member of the panel would even consider. But why is it so clear that these two alternatives exhaust the moral possibilities of the described case and that the path of direct termination is beyond the pale?

First of all, it is not clear that meningitis would be an efficient "friend." As Dr. Reich pointed out, babies have been known to survive the meningitis and live a number of years without being aware of anything and requiring a great amount of physical care. Thus the problem could be intensified by mere omission and reliance on the disease to achieve the desired results. Furthermore, as one of the doctors in the audience pointed out in this discussion, death by meningitis in such cases is not normally serene. Disease in this instance may not come to the aid of ethics.

There can be good reasons offered to keep a child like this alive. Advances are being made in the treatment of nearly all the symptoms of this affliction. It may even be argued that if people do not take a chance on life for such children, medicine will not be able to learn all that it needs to conquer and prevent this disorder. Caution is further indicated by the basic fact that a decision is being made for another person.

Given the realities of the case as described, however, it is possible that death might be seen as preferable to the kind of life this child could have. The moral question then is whether the death should be entrusted to the imminent disease or whether it could be brought on by the administration of drugs or whether a compromise could be found whereby the drugs are used to comfort and to weaken in coordination with the meningitis. In the current state of legal and moral debate, the latter possibility would offer the advantage of protective ambiguity. Still, this flight to ambiguity would represent a retreat from the question: Can it be moral and should it be legal to take direct action to terminate life in certain circumstances?

Another of the terrible new powers of medicine is its ability to prolong life at a vegetative level. Take the case of a patient whose spontaneous brain activities are limited to those arising from the brain stem which controls breathing and circulation. Such a creature can be kept alive with stimulants and nourishment for a long period of time. Does it make good sense to do so?

The determination of death twenty-five years ago was not a very difficult job. Today, the old criteria have been robbed of their simplicity. Prompt cardiac resuscitation can restore a normal heartbeat in many cases, and mechanical assistance can keep a heart going that has lost all spontaneous capacity to pump. In some cases, as we mentioned, the brain could be quite dead and yet respirators could keep cardiovascular and respiratory functions going.

An agreement on brain death might present itself as the obvious solution, but here, as anywhere, facile solutions are suspect. There is the practical problem of how to determine that a person is dead of brain and therefore dead. A flat EEG might seem to be a clear-cut criterion for brain death. It is not. Persons with flat EEG's for several hours have been known to recover. Furthermore, persons with flat EEG's have been observed to continue breathing for up to six hours. There are, however, other ways of supporting the judgment that death has overtaken the brain which medical science is exploring.

Dr. Julius Korein, professor of neurology at the New York University School of Medicine, distinguishes between brain death (death of the entire brain including brain stem) and cerebral death. He concludes that when cerebral death has been determined, the physician should pronounce the patient cerebrally dead and suggest the discontinuation of cardiovascular and pulmonary support systems. It is his opinion that "advances in medicine have accelerated development of techniques that will allow the physician to define and diagnose cerebral death with accuracy and rapidity in an appropriate hospital setting." If this is true, the concept of cerebral death may be the best that can be done by way of bringing up-to-date the detection of death.

But what of the organs of the cerebrally dead? If we pull the plugs and allow the patient to die fully — heart, lungs, and even brain stem — we might also have waited so long that asphyxia will have damaged all organs for potential transplant. In a case in which the heart is still beating by reason of brain stem functioning although cortical activity is entirely extinguished, could this patient be declared dead so as to make it possible to keep him (it) breathing for purposes of transfer of tissue? To tie the definition of death to the organ needs of others might build a conflict of interest in the medical profession which is not in the best interests of the departing patient. The specter of organ piracy might come to dwell over the deathbed. But if it can be seen that the cortically brain dead patient is departed, not departing, it should be possible to devise sufficient safeguards to ensure that organ needs do not hasten the declaration of death.

In a survey of 250 Chicago internists and surgeons, 156 responded to a questionnaire asking: "In your opinion do physicians actually practice euthanasia in instances of incurable adult sufferers?" Sixty-one percent affirmed that physicians actually practice it, at least by omission, or what is sometimes called passive euthanasia. What is most revealing, however, is that 72 percent said the practice should not be legalized. Thus, although it occurs, they think, in the practice of a majority of their colleagues, it should not be permitted.

Louis Lasagna, M.D., argues that decisions on lengthening or shortening life are unavoidable for doctors, and mentions a survey that shows that about a third of all doctors feel that mercy killing is justified in the case of a terminal patient who is in great pain without hope of relief or recovery. He adds that many physicians covertly practice euthanasia in the case of children born with gross congenital abnormalities by not resuscitating the child at birth.

Back in 1957, Pope Pius XII, no radical in the field of ethics, addressed the question of whether a respirator can be turned off if the patient is in a final and hopeless state of unconsciousness. The Pope reasoned that the respirator in these circumstances is not morally obligatory, and therefore it can be turned off. He recognized that this action causes "the arrest of circulation," but he said it is nonetheless licit.

Many American physicians feel that this position is reasonable and permissible under American law. Many more are not so sure, and one can sympathize with their uncertainty. Lawyer William Cannon considers the matter of "pulling the plug" under American law and comes up with this conclusion: "If it is concluded to be an omission, the law is murky at best. If, however, it is concluded to be an affirmative act, the law has a ready charge: Murder in the first degree."

Professor Bayless Manning is probably accurate when he says that "decisions are predominantly being made by thousands of doctors in millions of different situations and by undefined, particularized, *ad hoc* criteria." This state of affairs is not something desirable under law for it leaves things to the vagaries of a "rule of man" instead of providing for the fairness and consistency of a "rule of law."

# Health Occupations Credentialing: Three Views — A Report on SASHEP

*by William K. Selden, Don Frey and*

*Thomas Ginley*

**William K. Selden, LL.D., Litt.D.,** who contributed the section on A Report on SASHEP, is currently director, Study of Accreditation of Selected Health Educational Programs, sponsored by the American Medical Association, National Commission on Accrediting, and Association of Schools of Allied Health Professions. He also served as director of the study described here.

**Mr. Don Frey,** who contributed the section on A Look at Institutional Credentialing, is executive director of the Health careers Council of Illinois in Chicago.

**Dr. Thomas Ginley,** who contributed the section on The Accrediting Agency View, is with the American Dental Association's Council on Dental Education.

The Study of Accreditation of Selected Health Educational Programs (SASHEP) was initiated by the American Medical Association's Council on Medical Education and the Council's Advisory Committee for Allied Health Professions and Services. It was conducted on a cooperative basis with two other sponsors, the Association of Schools of Allied Health Professions and the National Commission on Accrediting, and a grant of approximately $240,000 from the Commonwealth Fund. We focused the study on 15 selected fields in which accreditation was then being conducted in collaboration with the AMA.

## Definitions

I would like to describe the definitions which we use regarding accreditation, certification, licensure, and registration. Even though most of you do have them clearly in mind, there may be some who are confused by the terms. *Accreditation* is the process by which an agency or organization evaluates and recognizes a program of study or an institution as meeting certain predetermined qualifications or standards. It shall apply only to institutions and their programs of study or their services.

*Certification* is the process by which a non-governmental agency or association grants recognition to an individual who has met certain predetermined qualifications established by that agency or association.

*Licensure* is the process by which a governmental agency grants permission to the persons meeting predetermined qualifications to engage in a given occupation and/or use a particular title, or grants permission to institutions to perform specified functions.

*Registration* is the process by which qualified individuals are listed on an official roster maintained by a governmental or nongovernmental agency.

Our study was specifically and directly concerned with the first of those — accreditation. The staff, comprising three individuals, prepared with two consultants a series of working papers, the main issues of which are summarized in the first section of the commission's final report.

The second section of the final report is entitled "Basic Policies for Accreditation." It was prepared because there were no such documents to which we could refer, and we believed that basic policies should be enunciated that

could be applied to all post-secondary education.

The third section contains three parts. The first part presents a series of alternatives to the current accreditation situation. The alternatives range all the way from discontinuing accreditation for all allied health programs, in favor of total reliance on certification or licensure, to supporting government regulations as an alternative to educational accreditation by a non-governmental agency.

The second part of section three comprises conclusions. These were an attempt to enunciate certain specific philosophical principles regarding the relationship and responsibilities of the health profession.

Part three contains specific recommendations for restructuring accreditation for the 15 fields studied. These recommendations have attracted the most attention. Little attention has been given to the more basic issues presented in the conclusions of part two, some of which I would like to present here.

Conclusion A. "When oriented toward the needs of society, specialized accreditation of health educational programs provides a necessary, vital service to society and should be therefore continued." As a commission we were convinced that in our society nongovernmental accreditation, oriented primarily for the need of society and not toward the protection of a particular profession, is a major means of providing surveillance and help, particularly in the health field.

## Interprofessional Relationships

Conclusion B. "Fundamental changes in the organization of accreditation of allied health educational programs are needed to promote improvement in interprofessional relationships; to provide greater assurance to society that the accrediting process will be conducted in the public interest; and to provide a more equitable balance among the many diverse parties having a legitimate interest in the accreditation of allied health educational programs." The organizations now taking action as a result of the report have not directed their attention to this particular segment, but have directed their attention toward the implementation methods that we have suggested. But it is the *acceptance* of these principles which is the important factor, and not specifically how they are implemented.

Conclusion B-1 touches a very sensitive nerve. "Physicians must be intimately involved in the process of accrediting programs of study in all of the selected allied health fields. However, the approval of standards and the accreditation of these programs of study must be subject to final authority of a body that represents no single profession." We are talking about issues in which there must be some give and take, an understanding of other points of view, and recognition of the historical development.

One more conclusion (B-2): "The accreditation of allied health educational programs must promote increased collaboration, cooperation, and coordination among the health profes-

sions." The accreditation of allied health educational programs must be organized to improve both its effectiveness and its efficiency.

This is just a sample of what we concluded in our study. There are several other points that I should mention. By the time our study was completed, the number of fields in which accreditation was being conducted on a collaborative basis for the final supervision of the AMA, had increased from 15 to 20. Six other organizations are currently seeking approval from the AMA for inclusion in this group.

I will further add that there are some within the 15 studied that indicated a strong desire to conduct their accreditation independently of the AMA. There are others which do not have and do not seek affiliation with the AMA. It is perhaps unfortunate that they want to be so independent, and that the AMA on occasion is somewhat recalcitrant about wanting to be in complete charge.

## Interrelated Activities

We often look at accreditation as though it were a distinct function from the other activities in what is commonly known as credentialing. Earlier, I defined certification, accreditation, and licensure. It is my view that we must not encompass these three in one small part, but as we review and analyze ways to improve any one of the three, or to make changes and adjustments, it is necessary for us to recognize that they are interrelated, and that changes in one will influence the others. All three, particularly accreditation and licensure, are conducted for the public welfare. That is their primary, not their sole, but their primary purpose.

If the health professions collectively cannot reconcile their differences on matters such as accreditation, the only alternative in our society is for the federal government to assume greater responsibility than most government officials wish to exercise or assume. We must recognize that as professions are constituted they do not represent the public. Society has accorded them certain prerogatives — accreditation, for example — for the betterment of the public. If these functions are not conducted with primary interest for the public welfare, then it is necessary for the government, which represents all of us, to bring in certain civil or political pressures which may or may not be existent in the present operation.

I say this with no idea of threat. I do not say it in a spirit of bemoaning what might happen, but within our society it is better for us to have a balance of forces which can be more effective if the private sector will collectively assume, with less rivalry, broader recognition of interprofessional responsibilities.

## A LOOK AT INSTITUTIONAL CREDENTIALING

Institutions in pursuit of a single objective called "patient care" employ a variety of specialists to achieve it, and the ways in which these personnel are credentialed by the institutions can affect education in the health field.

Too often, when we talk about institutions determining the qualifications of health personnel, it's received as if the institution is going to write somebody a license to practice outside that institution. I would not even make that statement except that, in discussing this over a period of years now, I have heard it repeatedly. Of course, each institution does have a valid interest in credentialing personnel for service within its own organizational framework. USOE has funded an experiment in institutional accrediting in Illinois, as called for in the 1971 Richardson Report.

### Compartmented System

From the managerial point of view, our present compartmented system of producing people for work in the health field doesn't offer very much flexibility. The idea of the "team" is honored more in language than in actuality, and separate departments in a hospital operate in many different ways, without necessarily relating to the whole patient.

In addition, the proliferation of specialization is leading to a situation where only specially trained technicians are allowed to perform certain narrowly defined functions. Obviously, this cannot continue, and it is one reason why some individuals have recently called for some national (if you will note, not "federal") system of credentialing.

A third point is economic determinism. Since 1940, when third party payers began to grow, the health service industry has been able to charge what it needed in order to perform its service. The health insurance company or other third party payer simply raised its rates, and that cycle went on week after week. But the government has become an increasing part of this third party payment, and that gravy train has come to an end. Third party payers, including the government, are asking how long we can go on subsidizing an industry just because it happens to operate in hundred-million-dollar institutions. Maybe we should look at what we are paying people to do, and whether they are overqualified, overpaid, or what have you. This, then, is another reason for looking at credentials and institutional credentialing.

A fourth, strong reason is a social one. Most health professionals come from middle class backgrounds. Many people who work in the health service industries have just as much potential but come from disadvantaged backgrounds and are hopelessly held down within the industry because of their inability to spend two, three, five, or maybe up to 15 years getting educated for professional positions. Yet many of them do get qualified through life experience education instead of formal education. It is time to halt the enormous and growing power that colleges and universities have as screening institutions, and the reliance on educational credentials as admission tickets to careers. We must develop mechanisms and criteria for measuring an individual's potential that are more relevant than those now universally recognized.

## Legal Aspects

The legal view of professional power is also a factor here. Many of the writers in this area, Nathan Hershey, for example, are lawyers. We have been interested in this in Illinois for quite a long time, and in 1965 we had a monumental case here, Darling *versus* Charleston Hospital.

A boy broke his leg in a football game and was taken to a local hospital where a doctor set his leg. Gangrene set in and his leg had to be amputated. It turned out that the doctor had only tried setting legs three times before and two of them had been unsuccessful. The nurses knew this leg was set wrong and said so, but were told to follow the doctor's orders. The nurses and the hospital used that as a defense, but the Supreme Court of the State of Illinois said no.

A hospital practices medicine, the Court said, and it is responsible for what goes on inside and should have rules. So the validity of the educational credentials of the individuals involved is the responsibility of the institution.

## Next Step

It is easy, from there, for an institution to say, "If we are responsible anyway, and we have to make a determination of whether or not someone is qualified, regardless of his educational preparation, then what difference does it make if he has a formal education? We can determine that ourselves."

The coronary care nurse who practices medicine and possibly surgery under existing rules in an institution is practicing something that she is not licensed to do. The commercial school graduate working side by side in a laboratory with an ASCP medical technologist may have acquired in some way or another parallel competencies, but only one of them has that credential. The hospital administrator doesn't have to have any credentials. I know a high school dropout who runs a 500-bed hospital. How did that board find out whether he was qualified?

The most obvious indication I know of institutional credentialing is the organized staff of any medical hospital. Physicians are licensed to practice medicine and surgery in all of its branches in the state of Illinois. That credential gets them into an organized hospital medical staff, then what they are allowed to do within that institution is determined by rules and criteria set up by its medical staff. If an individual proves to be incompetent on a continuing basis, the staff removes those privileges. So it has existed for a long time, in other industries as well as in health services.

## Quality Control

In a pharmaceutical house a high school dropout can compound a prescription. However, the pharmacist who pours this preparation into little bottles is under strict controls. Licensing is a quality control mechanism. Institutional credentialing shifts the responsibility for quality control to the institutions themselves.

This calls for a careful definition of the quality we are seeking to control. What *is* quality patient care or quality medical service? You must test your product against your definition, so job definition and description become essential.

This is where institutional credentialing will have its chief effect on education, because this determines the kind of products we are after in patient care. From this kind of job description, we can develop methods for measuring a person's qualifications for a job, and devise ways of providing students with skills they need to be "qualified."

## THE ACCREDITING AGENCY VIEW

This is an era of accountability and due process both in education and in accreditation. Although education has become more sensitive to both of these issues in the last few years, accrediting agencies have only recently been required to exercise similar concern.

As administrators of a specialized accrediting agency within the health field, we have become extremely sensitive to the various problems associated with specialized or professional accreditation. What, specifically, is the role of specialized accreditation? Generally, it is based on these premises:

A. There is a demand for the services of a given occupation or vocation.

B. There is a need to determine the educational program necessary for preparing the occupational or vocational practitioner.

21

C. The identification of the educational qualifications related to program development is a *shared responsibility* between educational institutions and professionals within the field associated with the occupation.

D. Appropriate specialized agencies or associations are in the best position to offer institutional guidance, provide educational standards development and meaningful input into educational institutions that are developing programs according to established criteria.

E. The public is entitled to know which institutions offer acceptable training in a given vocation or occupation.

Clearly, these ideas are interrelated and have developed an immense enterprise of specialized and professional accreditation. This growth, however, has not been without its difficulties.

As Dr. Selden indicates in the SASHEP report, specialized accreditation, when properly oriented, provides an invaluable service to society that perhaps cannot be duplicated through any other procedure. Although there is evidence to suggest that that statement is true, it should not be interpreted to signify that accreditation, on the basis of its current status, has been without its critics or that accreditation has been equally responsive to society.

## Positive Influence

Rather, accreditation should be viewed as a positive influence which at the present time may not have fulfilled all of its expectations. Accreditation, because of its proliferation, has inadvertently become the target for many of the problems associated with education. Admittedly, many of the expressed concerns are accurate. Quoting again from the SASHEP Commission report, I cannot help but concur with a comment by Quigg Newton, president of the Commonwealth Fund, concerning the grant award for the conduct of the SASHEP study.

"Professional education in these fields — which have become an increasingly vital component of the nation's health services — is being seriously encumbered by the costly maze of accreditation requirements and procedures imposed by the multiplicity of professional associations that characterize this important health man-power sector.

"The public interest requires that a means be found to promote collaboration between professional associations in allied health and educational institutions in these fields in an effort to create a new system of accreditation that will make possible a coherent, flexible, and rational approach to manpower development."

## Cumulative Concern

While it should be noted that this comment related to the development of a study for selected allied health professional programs, the statement basically can be applied to all forms of specialized or professional accreditation. Although accreditation may be viewed as a singular activity of the agencies responsible for conducting it, it is clearly a cumulative concern from the institution's point of view.

A specialized or professional accrediting agency may indeed consider its mission as valuable to society and to the institution, and there is probably justification for both opinions. One must also view with some concern the direction and significance being placed on accreditation by non-educational sectors, such as government and society in general. Clearly, other functions or uses for accreditation procedures have been added to the original purpose.

Accreditation has been defined as simply a process whereby an organization or agency recognizes an educational program of study as having met certain predetermined qualifications or standards. While this simple definition conjures up an endless array of questions, the intent of the definition is fairly clear.

As I see it, specialized and professional accreditation is on a collision course with the demands of society, the changing role of educational institutions, the demands of government and, quite pragmatically, the financial capability of institutions to meet the demands of accrediting agencies. Although I am a representative of a specialized accrediting agency, one must take the position of devil's advocate occasionally and admit that there is a real world beyond the confines of a special interest area. Nevertheless, it is clear that we still must resist the potential demise of voluntary accreditation in the United States. At the present time, accreditation is in desperate need of a voluntary agency to control its future.

## Regulating Accreditation Agencies

Many of you are perhaps aware of the respective roles of the U.S. Office of Education and the National Commission on Accrediting in regulating, to some degree, the accrediting activities of regional, specialized, and professional agencies in the United States. In recent years, USOE has become increasingly prominent in the field of accrediting agency review. Currently it is necessary for an accrediting agency to gain recognition and undergo periodic review by USOE and the national Commission on Accrediting to determine continued eligibility to function as a recognized accrediting agency in the United States.

Criteria have been established which must be met by the individual accrediting agency in order to secure this recognition. The criteria used by USOE to recognize accrediting agencies are, in my view, sound and have as their primary motive a goal shared by the National Commission on Accrediting (and hopefully by all specialized and professional accrediting agencies), i.e., the improvement of the educational process through better accreditation procedures.

In recent years, some have become skeptical and critical of the increasing role of the U.S. Office of Education in the affairs of accreditation. I, for one, shared that concern, yet realize now that USOE's motives are sound and are simply being developed because we, as voluntary accrediting agencies, have been remiss in a part of our function and perhaps have to some degree violated a trust granted by society.

This, of course, is the hard view of our existence and what must be understood by all of us is that the criticisms can no longer be ignored but must be dealt with in an intelligent manner. A government agency has begun to indicate the way to go. Guidelines are there and they demonstrate the critical need for a strong spokesman and regulator for voluntary accreditation in these United States.

## Integrating Accreditation

The intent of these comments is to direct the consideration of the credentialing process, from the viewpoint of specialized accrediting agencies, to indicate the changes necessary to sustain some reasonableness and value for accreditation. With this theme as a basis, I suggest the need — and I am convinced there is an urgency associated with it — for a strong agency to be developed through the proposed merger of the National Commission on Accrediting and the Federation of Regional Accrediting Commissions of Higher Education.

While this organization should include specialized and professional accrediting agencies as well as appropriate public members, the agency should not simply be a spokesman or agency of our specialized interests. Rather, it must be developed into the mechanism which regulates and controls all voluntary accreditation in the United States.

I can see no way short of such a system — with the exception of federal government accreditation and review — which will eventually allow the integration of all accreditation. Further, agencies may have to adjust their parochial interests to allow for greater cooperation and coordination of accrediting activities. Specialized accrediting agencies may have to modify their structure and function to allow for greater input from all affected groups. It may be tradition which allows only the chief professional agency in a multi-disciplined field to have the overall responsibility for development and approval of educational standards and the actual accreditation process, but in this era of accountability the procedure will have to be modified to include other appropriate representatives.

In the final analysis, independent specialized accreditation can no longer exist in a vaccum and what is being asked of us by others is no more than we should ask of ourselves — reasonableness in the affairs of accreditation.

*Reprinted with permission
from* Saturday Review,
Vol. I, No. 2 (March 1973) page 22.
Copyright by
Saturday Review Company March 1973.

# The Patient's Bill of Rights

## Willard Gaylin

*On January 8 of this year the American Hospital Association published a "Patient's Bill of Rights," covering what the association calls the most commonly questioned situations that patients encounter in a hospital. In the following guest editorial, Dr. Willard Gaylin, cofounder and president of the Institute of Society, Ethics and the Life Sciences in Hastings-on-Hudson, New York, argues that the prerogative to define patients' rights lies elsewhere.*

*Willard Gaylin, M.D.*, is currently President of the Institute of Society, Ethics and the Life Sciences in Hastings-on-Hudson, New York.

A stay in a hospital exposes an individual to a condition of passivity and impotence unparalleled in adult life, this side of prison. You are dressed in an uncomfortable garment, leaving you exposed and ludicrous; told when you must sleep and when you must rise; informed of what you may eat and when you have to eat it; notified as to when you can have visitors, who they shall be, and how long they can stay. You are discussed in the third person in your presence as though you were some idiot child or inanimate object. If you are unfortunate enough to have an interesting case, you will be presented to a group of strangers who may take the invasion of your privacy as their privilege. Your chart, at the foot of the bed, will contain all the vital information that you would seem to be entitled to have; yet, should you attempt to examine it, you will be treated like a prepubescent caught with a copy of *Portnoy's Complaint*.

Some of this may be necessary for health and some for convenience, but most of it is simply the inevitable result of an authoritative person dealing with people who unquestionably accept his authority.

Hospital regulations are endured by a patient conditioned to seeing his physician as a benevolent father in whose reassuring presence he is prepared to play the role of the child. Beyond this, however, more serious rights are violated under the numbing atmosphere of the same paternalism.

Modern scientific medicine, as exemplified in complex teaching hospitals, has advanced technical skill at the cost of personal warmth. Often there is no one physician rendering care, rather a battery of specialists, and while "treatment" may be superior, "care" is absent. This depersonalization of medicine is having a predictable effect on the patient, causing him to abandon his tendency to romanticize the physician, and, by extension, the medical community. For this and other reasons the patient is now pressing for a reevaluation of the medical contract.

In response to this, the American Hospital Association recently presented, with considerable fanfare, a "Patient's Bill of Rights." It is a document worth examining, for nothing indicates the low estate of current hospital care (as distinguished from treatment) more graphically than the form of the proffered cure.

The substance of the document is amazingly innocent of controversy. It affirms that "the patient has the right to considerate and respectful care" and, beyond that, the right to "reasonable continuity of care."

He is told that he may expect a modicum of personal privacy; that the usual medical concern for confidentiality should be respected; that he has a right to expect "a reasonable response" to his request for service; and, as in any other commercial transaction, that he has a right to receive an explanation of his bill.

In addition, he will be relieved to hear that, as a patient in a hospital, knowledge of the "rules and regulations" that apply to him is manifestly his due—just as it would be if he were a participant in a poker game. Similarly, the right to obtain information "concerning his diagnosis, treatment and prognosis" seems perfectly straightforward—no more than the minimum required of any standard commercial transaction. On the other hand, the patient's right to "obtain information as to any relationship of his hospital to other health care and educational institutions in so far as his care is concerned" is disquieting, for it anxiously suggests that while his exclusive reason for being in the hospital is his personal health, the hospital may have multiple, unstated other reasons influencing its treatment of him.

Finally, when the bill affirms the patient's right to "give informed consent prior to the start of any procedure," his "right to refuse treatment to the extent permitted by law," and his right to be advised "if the hospital proposes to engage in or perform human experimentation" on him, it seems to be merely belaboring the obvious. It says no more than that the hospital is subject to the same laws concerning assault and battery as any other institution or member of society.

The objection to this well-intended, though timid, document is that it perpetuates the very paternalism that precipitated the abuses. By presenting its considerations as a "Patient's Bill of Rights," it creates the impression that the hospital is "granting" these rights to the patient. The hospital has no power to grant these rights. They were vested in the patient to begin with. If the rights have been violated, they have been violated by the hospital and its hirelings. The title a "Patient's Bill of Rights" therefore seems not only pretentious but deceptive. In effect, all that the document does is return to the patient, with an air of largess, some of the rights hospitals have previously stolen from him. It is the thief lecturing his victim on self-protection—i.e., the hospital instructs the patient to make sure that the hospital treats him according to the rules of decency and law to which he is entitled. It would be more appropriate if the association addressed its 7,000 member hospitals, cautioning them that for years they have violated patient rights, some of which have the mandate of law, and warning them they must no longer presume on the innocence of their customers or the indifference of judicial authorities.

Since this is a patently decent document, the fact that the American Hospital Asssociation takes the circuitous route of speaking to the patient of his rights, rather than to the hospital of its duties, reveals the essential weakness of such professional organizations. The AHA, like the American Medical Association and similar groups, is designed to be the servant of its constituent members—and not of the general public. A servant does not lay down the law to his master. In this regard the AHA can only state that it "presents these rights in the expectation that they will be supported" by the member hospitals. The fact that it feels the need to alert the patient indicates how insecure that "expectation" is.

A reevaluation of patient rights —one that goes beyond the old rights reaffirmed in this bill—is greatly needed. The public should not look to the professional association for leadership here. It is not for the hospital community to outline the rights it will offer, but rather for the patient consumer to delineate and then demand those rights to which he feels entitled, by utilizing all the instruments of society designed for that purpose—including the legislature and the courts.

Rapid changes in nursing practice create demands for continuing education. It is a truism that "nursing just isn't like it used to be" and that some form of continuing education is imperative for professional practice. Most nurses accept this, but the debate is over the best way to assure professional competency.

# *Continuing education should be voluntary*

## *Signe S. Cooper*

**Signe S. Cooper, R.N., M.Ed.** is professor of nursing and chairman, Department of Nursing, University of Wisconsin Extension, Madison, Wisconsin. She is also chairman of the interim executive committee, Council on Continuing Education, American Nurses' Association.

*Definitions.* "Continuing education" in the broadest sense includes all those learning activities that occur beyond the basic preparatory program; in the case of nursing, it is the education following that leading to initial licensure to practice.

Continuing education is *not* primarily credit courses toward a degree, although such courses are often acceptable in meeting requirements for recognition systems established by state nurses' associations. Thus, our present systems of nursing education includes three major components: basic, graduate, and continuing education.

The terms *inservice education* and *continuing education* are not synonymous. Inservice education is that provided by an employing agency for its employees; is related specifically to job improvement; and is part of an individual's continuing education. Inservice education is often acceptable to meet part of the requirements for recognition systems of continuing education and certain aspects may be acceptable for meeting legal requirements as they are established, but some segments, such as orientation to a specific institution, will not be acceptable.

Continuing education includes more than formal courses, and often definitions of continuing education place too much emphasis on formal course work. Each of us learns in his own way, and we select those ways most useful to us. Some of these approaches to learning, such as reading and library study, discussion with colleagues about a nursing care problem, or other independent study methods may not be acceptable for meeting continuing education requirements.

It is possible to learn a great deal on the job—particularly if we *plan* to learn. Some aspects of employment may be viewed as continuing education, but it may be difficult to make clear-cut distinctions between enriching work experiences and those that result in minimal learning.

For the nurse who claims to be a professional, continuing education must be broader than merely those aspects that relate to a specific job; it must include content of significance to the nursing profession generally. The nurse must not only have knowledge of various aspects of nursing, but must be familiar with current developments in nursing. For example, she must have at least some knowledge of the difference between a clin-

ical nurse practitioner and a clinical nurse specialist; an awareness of the report of the National Commission on Nursing and Nursing Education; a familiarity with various aspects of the current issues in nursing. One of these issues relates to mandatory continuing education. To date, California and New Mexico have established continuing education requirements for relicensure to practice nursing. Several other states have similar legislation pending.

*"Continuing education must be broader than merely those aspects that relate to a specific job."*

In contrast to the mandatory approach, continuing education is often *voluntary*. This may be viewed in three different ways. First, there is education in which we participate by our own choice.

Another voluntary approach is the recognition systems established by several state nurses' associations. When certain previously established requirements have been met, the nurse is provided a document which recognizes this achievement. Although not required as a condition of membership, the majority of members participate in their associations' recognition systems.

Sometimes organizations require continuing education as a condition of membership. However, this could still be viewed as voluntary continuing education, since membership in the association is voluntary.

*Arguments against mandatory continuing education.* The arguments against requiring continuing education as a condition for relicensure for nursing are both practical and philosophical. The practical arguments, which relate primarily to resources, may not be uniformly applicable, but the philosophical arguments have broad application.

*Practical reasons.* The major practical argument against mandatory continuing education is lack of adequate educational resources. Until fairly recently, only sporadic interest was shown in the provision of continuing education for nurses on a systematic basis. Since there are not enough education resources available to meet the wide variety of educational needs of nurses, establishing mandatory requirements may create hardships for some nurses, particularly those who live outside metropolitan areas.

With limited resources, nurses may enroll in workshops or short courses not suited to their learning needs only to meet the licensure requirement. Under these circumstances, establishing mandatory requirements creates hostility and resentment—attitudes which interfere with learning.

A second practical argument relates to the problems of accrediting or approving suitable offerings. When continuing education is required by legislation, some means of official approval must be established for available learning experiences. At present, boards of nursing are neither prepared nor staffed to accredit the available continuing education offerings, let alone additional ones that may be established to meet requirements.

A third practical argument against mandatory continuing education relates to evaluation. To date, tools for measuring the effectiveness of continuing education are inadequate. There are few definitive studies showing the positive effects of continuing education on the improvement of nursing care. Such research in continuing education will be further delayed as pressures are placed on potential researchers to provide more educational offerings.

Given enough time, money, and prepared teachers, the obstacles in these practical arguments could eventually be overcome. However, the philosophical arguments are more significant than are the practical reasons.

*Philosophical arguments.* By their very nature, legal requirements tend to be inflexible and rigid. As important as legal requirements were for upgrading the quality of schools of nursing, they led to conformity among the schools and inhibited experimentation in nursing curricula.

Some of the critical problems faced by the nursing profession today relate to the education of nurses in the past, and the inflexibility of schools of nursing to meet the needs of a changing society.

Legal requirements must be quite specific to achieve their purposes and to be fair to all concerned. If they are too flexible, they are impossible to monitor. Thus, it is a paradox to talk about flexible requirements. The advocates of mandatory continuing education use the argument that there are many educational resources available: workshops, conferences, television, to name a few. Yet without adequate testing, it is impossible to measure the extent of the learning that results from participation in these activities. Without some means of measurement, it seems pointless to recognize these learning activities for legal purposes, even though no one would deny their educational value to the individual learner.

*"When continuing education is compulsory for relicensure, we are denying the nurse's professionalism . . ."*

Rigid legal requirements do not allow for individual differences in learning. Establishing legal requirements downgrades professional autonomy and the right of the individual to decide which learning approaches are best suited to his needs.

Just when it appears that nursing has achieved some autonomy, the proposed action for licensure requirements will negate it. When continuing education is compulsory for relicensure, we are denying the nurse's professionalism—someone else is deciding what she needs to know.

The nursing profession needs independent thinkers and motivated, self-directed learners. Fostering dependency on the educational system is not the way to achieve this goal. The excitement of learning is rarely fostered in an environment of forced participation.

*"A positive approach would be for nurses to begin now to assess their own learning needs, exploring available resources . . ."*

Legal requirements are always minimal requirements. Once these requirements have been met, there is a tendency to discontinue learning activity until the next relicensure period, rather than recognize that learning is a continuous process.

You really cannot force people to learn. In our system of general education, we have legislated the amount of time that people spend in the classroom, but we cannot legislate the learning that occurs there. Recognizing the futility of compulsory education laws for some students, legislation has been introduced in Wisconsin to lower the age of compulsory school attendance.

The most significant argument against mandatory continuing education may be that it fosters negative attitudes toward learning, and thus results in less learning by the individual than would otherwise occur.

*Alternatives to mandatory continuing education.* It seems obvious that if nurses had accepted a personal responsibility for lifelong learning for professional practice, we would not be in our present position. The push for mandatory continuing education has resulted, in large measure, from the concerns of consumers for a better quality of care. The assumption that continuing education will result in better care is yet to be proved.

A positive approach would be for nurses to begin now to assess their own learning needs, explore available resources for continuing their education, and take advantage of them. Thus, the most reasonable alternative is that of individual acceptance of the personal responsibility for continued learning.

Professional certification seems a more logical approach to determining competence than establishing mandatory continuing education requirements. The recent announcement by the American Nurses' Association of its nationwide certification program to recognize excellence in the clinical practice of nursing is of particular significance.

Peer review has been suggested as another alternative. To be effective, peer review takes considerable skill and objectivity, and it may be some time before many nurses are ready for this type of sophisticated evaluation. Nevertheless, attempts at peer review are being initiated in a few places.

Another alternative is that of voluntary systems tied to the professional association. Such plans are underway in many of the state nurses' associations and other organizations, and have been described in the nursing literature.

*"For a number of reasons, mandatory continuing education is no guarantee of competency to practice."*

Maintaining the competency of practitioners is one of the most critical problems relating to the delivery of health care. Consumers expect health professionals to maintain their competency, and their demands for competent practice have resulted in proposals for mandatory continuing education as one condition for relicensure.

For a number of reasons, mandatory continuing education is no guarantee of competency to practice. The effective nurse will accept a personal responsibility for maintaining competency, and recognize that participating in continuing education will assist the process.

# Mandatory Continuing Education for Nurses

*Erline P. McGriff*

**Erline Perkins McGriff, R.N., Ed.D.,** is professor and head, Division of Nursing, School of Education, Health, Nursing, and Arts Professions, New York University.

Continuing education in nursing may be defined as those planned learning experiences which are designed for nurses, members of other health disciplines, and consumers of health care services. Its focus would be directed toward developing greater community awareness among nurses and toward strengthening community and inter-disciplinary participation in planning and implementing health services for all people. An interdisciplinary approach to continuing education in nursing explores ways in which nursing practice and the development of new nursing knowledge are related to members of other health groups and to consumers of health care to improve the nature and delivery of health care services.

33

*"Nursing must move ahead in support of the principle of mandatory continuing education for nurses."*

*Continuing Education for nurses.* Continuing education for nurses must focus primarily on those learning experiences which relate directly to the practice and scope of nursing. It may be defined as those learning activities which occur after an individual has completed a basic nursing education program. This definition would apply to licensed or vocational nurses. The concept of continuing education should be inherent in any basic educational program. Nurses must establish an early commitment to a career of lifelong learning.

The contemporary knowledge explosion, technological advances, and public demands for more effective health services make it imperative that nurses continue their learning beyond the formal education process.

These factors make it impossible for any nurse to expect, or to be expected, to carry on a successful career without further learning. Keeping up-to-date is a demanding task for all who nurse; for those who must exercise leadership in developing new approaches to the nature and delivery of health services, the demands are greater.

*Who is responsible for continuing education?* Efforts towards assessing needs, planning, and implementing successful programs in continuing education in nursing and for nurses require input from a variety of sources. All efforts should be consumer-oriented.

There are four groups which may be identified as having responsibilities. They are: 1) educational institutions; 2) employers of nurses; 3) professional and other organizations; and 4) practitioners of nursing.

*Educational institutions.* Included under the umbrella of educational institutions are community colleges, senior colleges, and universities. Each has a signal responsibility to plan, develop, and implement programs in continuing education. Each one should determine what it can do best to avoid duplication of effort among institutions. Educational institutions must move into leadership positions since it is within such settings that nursing knowledge and related areas will be developed and renewed.

*Employers of nurses.* Employers of nurses must recognize their responsibility to facilitate participation of nurses in continuing education activities and programs. Such participation must extend beyond those responsibilities that all employers have for providing inservice education within any health care agency.

> *". . . This is the intent*
> *and the rationale*
> *on which a mandatory*
> *system . . . is based."*

> *"Continuing education*
> *for nurses is now,*
> *and always has been,*
> *voluntary."*

Some concrete avenues for facilitating nurses' participation in continued learning activities include: tuition remission plans; other policies regarding financial assistance; and provision for educational or sabbatical leaves. Suggestions have also been made to include in the personnel policies an accrual of "education days" comparable to the present practice of sick and other leave days. When employers possess a philosophical and financial commitment to continuing education, then it is not difficult to justify such efforts.

*Professional and other organizations.* Opportunities for continued learning through activities offered by professional and other organizations are almost innumerable. Such efforts need not be restricted to nursing groups, but must also include health, educational, and other related groups. Heart associations, regional medical programs, governmental agencies, diabetic associations, the National Health Council, and many others offer and provide rich resources for keeping up-to-date in specific areas of interest and importance.

*Practitioners of nursing.* The responsibility for providers of health care to keep up with current knowledge and practice must be seen as a personal commitment in which nurses remain accountable to consumers for quality health care services.

*The need to mandate continuing education for nurses.* Individual states need strong support to take a positive stand *for* mandatory continuing education in nursing as one condition for re-registration.

There is much misunderstanding about mandatory continuing education for nurses. Nurses must know that their initial license to practice will *not be revoked* if continuing education requirements are not met. It is the re-registration of that initial license which is affected.

There are forces outside of nursing which are indeed trying to eliminate individual licensure. Such forces include a movement toward medical certification and recommendations to eliminate State Boards of Nursing. Could there be a better reason for nurses to unite to retain authority over their responsibilities; to decide what nursing is; and then to do it? Nurses, however, cannot be satisfied until individual licensure measures up to its purported meaning, and this is the rationale on which a mandatory system for continuing education in nursing is based.

Nurses must also know that they will not be required to write another licensing examination; no nurse will be required to pursue an academic degree or go to college; and many activities will be considered to qualify for mandatory continuing education.

What about those nurses who engage in endeavors which do not include the direct practice of nursing? As long as these nurses choose to represent themselves as licensed practitioners of nursing, then they must give evidence that they meet the continuing education requirements for renewal of the initial license to practice nursing.

Activities which should qualify for meeting mandatory continuing education requirements are: courses taken for credit; non-credit courses; in-service education; refresher courses; independent methods of study (home study, programmed instruction, computer-assisted instruction, and self-directed study such as selected work experiences in the clinical practice of nursing); telephone-radio conferences; audio and video tapes and other recordings (cassettes); television programs and conferences; program meetings of professional and other organizations (clinical sessions); workshops; lectures; symposia; presentation and/or publication of scientific papers; correspondence courses; and other planned learning experiences or activities. Needless to say, a system of measurement must be adopted and adapted for approving such offerings. In addition, approval *in advance* of the offering is desirable.

Such an exhaustive list refutes the argument about the unavailability and inaccessibility of learning experiences for nurses. It also illustrates how mandatory requirements can meet the diverse continuing education needs of practicing nurses. Such varied offerings also account for individual differences in learning and in the learners.

As long weekends, longer vacation periods, shorter work weeks, and earlier retirements become a reality, the possibilities for nurses to be more creative in planning and responding to their own learning needs are enhanced.

Another major criticism of the mandatory concept has been that such a system does not recognize that one learns while "on the job." To ignore the fact that many nurses learn on an independent basis would be folly. However, to accept the premise that all one needs to know to keep up-to-date can be learned within one's "normal" work experience is likewise foolish. Such a belief is in conflict with the total concept of continuing education.

Some believe that continuing education for the professional should be voluntary, and that members of the professions are motivated to participate because of their deep sense of ethics and professional responsibility. Such is not the case. Nurses have historically believed that their basic educational programs in nursing prepared them for a lifetime of practice. The majority have not accepted the fact that nursing education is a continuous process.

Another criticism of the mandatory approach has been that "forcing" nurses to participate in a required number of learning activities may not result in learning. I would ask, "Has there ever been a guarantee that any learner will learn when exposed to a learning activity?"

While more learning may occur when incentives are internal (motivation) rather than external (which mandatory education would be), one cannot completely discount the effectiveness of learning with external incentives. Inattentiveness and resistance to learning are not necessarily related to external requirement. Internal requirements may also produce the same results.

To establish requirements for a mandatory system of continuing education for nurses, there has to be an effective relationship worked out between State Nurses' Associations and State Boards of Nursing. It is recommended that the operational framework for determining the validity of continuing education activities be the legal definition of nursing contained in the Nurse Practice Acts in each state.

State Nurses' Associations should assume leadership for approval of learning experiences according to criteria set by the professional association. State Boards of Nursing assume their responsibility for legal accountability to the nurse and to the public in re-registering those nurses who have met said requirements.

The time is past when a nurse who is a wife, mother, and homemaker can exempt herself from keeping informed professionally because "the effort required may be too taxing." When nurses examine their roles and responsibilities in the health care system it is evident that they will require continuing education. The crux of the matter may not really be whether continuing education for nurses will become mandatory—but rather who will *control* continuing education for nurses and indeed, nursing practice?

# NURSING EDUCATION AND PRACTICE:
# PUTTING IT ALL TOGETHER

### By Myrtle K. Aydelotte

The health delivery system in this country is undergoing closer scrutiny than ever before. This examination has been described by some writers as an attack; by others, as a rich opportunity for remodeling the system.

In these writings there are four central issues and concerns: the nature and characteristics of the roles for which professionals are prepared, especially that of the physician; the inequitable distribution of services provided to our population; the cost of health services; and the failure of the system

itself to be effective and sensitive. And there is a growing awareness of a need for the professionals to practice what is relevant to the client, rather than what enhances their own image. Unwillingness to accept accountability to clients, failures to meet health requirements of poor, black, and other minority groups, and a general inability to make health services accessible to all have been described and deplored. There is a swelling demand to reorient services from the delivery of a technical product to the provision

Myrtle K. Aydelotte, Ph.D., is director of Nursing, University of Iowa Hospitals and Clinics, and professor, College of Nursing.

Condensed from the Journal of Nursing Education, Vol. 11, Number 4, November 1972, Copyright © 1972 by McGraw-Hill.

of a social and personalized service to people.

Accomplishing these ends is dependent, in large part, upon the willingness and success with which recommendations of the Commission on Nursing and Nursing Education are carried out.

Nursing must examine the purpose for professional preparation. This purpose evolves from needs of people for specific human services. Society assigns to nursing assessment of patient wants and needs, design and execution of care practices; and instruction of patients and others in health maintenance, disease prevention, and aspects of care. Society allocates resources to prepare nurses who are sensitive to patient's wants, comprehensive procedures, technology and the behavioral and physical sciences that provide a basis of judgment.

There is great concern among some nurses over status, prestige, and control of programs, people, and decisions; more concern that nursing and nurses receive recognition than that they earn it. Although discrimination against nursing and nurses is well documented, one cannot ignore the lack of scholarship among faculty and ineffective nursing practice leadership, especially in matters of policy direction.

There are a few delivery systems demonstrating innovative and creative approaches to patient needs and there is some evidence of growing scholarship and statesmanship in nursing.

However, most directors of nursing services operate under traditional structures, policies, procedures, and practice roles which give strong evidence that imagination either lags or is missing. In many places, faculty members have virtually withdrawn from practice settings and are no longer seen as persons knowledgeable about nursing care. They perform ritualistic functions in sterile environments, perceiving themselves not as nurses but as educationists. They have severely limited interactions with clients, health professionals, and individuals who are attempting to make delivery systems function.

One group of nurse leaders lives in a world of tradition, anti-intellectualism, and blind acceptance of constraints; another group is shrouded in myths about what constitutes effective practice and is ignorant or denies constraints that are real and must be dealt with in the delivery of practice. The client and the new graduate are lost between these two worlds.

Nursing leadership must reorient itself and restructure itself in such a way that nursing education and practice are inseparable, are symbolic, and united in purpose. It must put aside inertia, apathy, competitiveness, personal animosities, and censorship. If it does not do this, society will surely place the charge it has given to nursing elsewhere.

Joining nursing education and practice tests professional leadership. Success depends upon four features:

1. Faculty research and experiments in practice settings in order to find what is relevant, effective, and economical in total patient care.
2. Clinical leadership in all delivery systems, regardless of setting, creating a new climate which responds to clients' needs and wants more effectively.
3. Allowing students and beginning practitioners to make their own connections between theory and application, with the help of articulated interaction between teachers and clinicians.
4. Nursing education and nursing practice establishing relationships that support and enhance each other, that make sense to the public, and that enable people to develop clinical leadership and participation in decisions affecting the national health system.

In my opinion, change must occur rapidly in the practice setting. Unless nursing leadership recognizes the importance of clinical care delivery, other major movements will be delayed. Many educators acknowledge this, but few contribute time and talent to the problems of remodeling the locus where students learn, graduates struggle, and research questions are generated. A few institutions are testing new models: Vanderbilt University; Case Western Reserve and University Hospitals of Cleveland; St. Luke's Presbyterian, Chicago; the University of Rochester; Providence General Hospital, Providence, Rhode Island; Good Samaritan Hospital, Phoenix.

What is needed are additional hospital and nonacute facility models in rural settings and small community agencies, testing and reporting the impact of change in practice upon the health of clients.

Faculty members, including Deans, must help in finding staff. Highly competent graduates must be encouraged to go into the delivery care system. Clinical Directors of Nursing must identify and evaluate patient care requirements in precise terms that are supported by hard data, use research findings in decision making, and plan purposeful programs. Unless close collaboration and mutual endorsement of goals are achieved by those in clinical nursing positions and in nursing education leadership positions, diffusion of purpose and direction, fragmentation of effort, and dislocation of people will occur in the health structure of the community.

Examples are now found in nursing literature, describing the role of clinicians and their contribution to patient care. Unfortunately, more attention is given to practitioner functions than to knowledge base or to the relationship of clinicians to faculty members and physicians.

Articles also describe attempts to build accountability to the client into various nursing roles. But these seem to be about alternatives on a theme rather than about fundamental changes by individual nurse practitioners. Perhaps the problems are not only those of personal resources and energy, but also conceptual. Remodeling of delivery systems should be directed toward individual care for the patient and the continuity of that care; not the continuity of *a nurse or other person* unless a one-to-one relationship in the provision of that service is documented as part of the therapy. It may well be that wholly unique patterns of assignment and staffing are indicated.

Several places are testing the primary care assignment, especially where a new role is introduced, such as the Pediatric Nurse Practitioner, the Family Nurse Practitioner, the Midwife, and the Nurse Clinician. It may be that the positions are too new to pose problems at the moment, but little has been said about the constraints which exist. Although one of the advantages suggested for these roles is the freedom to make decisions, the disadvantages of isolation, role ambiguity, financial constraints, questionable effectiveness, and sheer pressure of demands are not discussed freely. Follow-through on the recommendation of the National Commission concerning the establishment of joint practice commissions at a state level may assist in resolution of some problems and confusion.

Another study reports the problems of acceptance of the new practitioner, by physicians and by the nursing staff, but what happens to the patients when, and if, the practitioner leaves? One wonders if programmed care is the basis for introduction of new positions or whether the question is merely that of finding places in which to fit practioners. In order to bring about change in the care of clients, the purpose of the care program, the elements composing it, the phasing, and the evaluation plan should be laid prior to the implementation of new roles.

The Commission makes specific recommendations about nursing practice, clinical leadership, and the changing systems. Limited dialogue between the two types of leadership has been evident at national-level meetings. More and sustained dialogue should take place immediately, for these two groups must put the "nursing house" in order.

Reprinted with permission from *Journal of Obstetric, Gynecologic and Neonatal Nursing,* Volume 2, Number 5, (September-October, 1973), pp. 54–55.

# The New Morality Ethics and Nursing

*Louise B. Tyrer and William A. Granzig*

**Louise B. Tyrer, M.D., F.A.C.O.G.** is project director of the Division of Family Planning for The American College of Obstetricians and Gynecologists.

**William A. Granzig, Ph.D.** is administrator of the Physical Education Department of The American College of Obstetricians and Gynecologists and a lecturer in the Graduate School of Loyola University.

*The legalization of abortion and sterilization have forced many nurses to make additional decisions on ethical conduct. Such decisions cannot be based on scientific evidence and may be difficult for those trained as empiricists. "Laws" of ethics and morality are really "opinions," and nurses, patients, and others have the right to hold divergent beliefs. This right is asserted in NAACOG's Statement on Abortions and Sterilizations.*

With a change in the laws of many states concerning abortion and sterilization, many nurses are confronted with the necessity of making additional ethical decisions. Medicine and nursing are two disciplines that of necessity are based on scientific methods which generally call for the use of absolutes in dealing with health problems. Ethics, however, refer to the direction of conduct and to the guidance of the human act and are not absolute. Ethical decisions are based on the question: What should I do? These decisions are sometimes more difficult because they are based on custom or manner and vary from society to society.[1]

The nurse who attempts to use only her scientific training to determine ethical conduct will be in a quandary because seldom is there empirical evidence available to support her decision—no matter what it is. It is from nonscientific disciplines such as philosophy or theology that ethical decisions emanate. Some of these ethical or moral decisions are so highly valued by a society that they are structured into the legal code. These moral decisions that are governed by law have such a high societal value that a form of punishment is prescribed for anyone who violates them.

In a democratic society certain behaviors are left to the individual to decide. The truth of these decisions cannot be proven or disproven empirically, but nevertheless, they are held firmly and in some cases viewed as absolute truths. Pluralistic societies such as the United States allow for some divergence of beliefs in ethics and morality. One of the conditions of this freedom is that no one be forced into decisions that violate his or her ethical standards or, conversely, that no one force his or her own ethical beliefs on someone else.[2]

At present, some nurses feel that an ethical question arises in performing nursing duties for patients receiving abortion or sterilization services. While the society has not legislated against performing these services, a nurse may feel that assisting in providing care for patients undergoing abortion or sterilization procedures is a clear violation of her ethical standards. The nurse is troubled by the "What should I do?" of her conscience.

In an attempt to aid the nurse facing this ethical question, the Nurses Association of The American College of Obstetricians and Gynecologists approved on May 31, 1972, a statement on abortion and sterilization, which is printed in full below:

> The Nurses Association of The American College of Obstetricians and Gynecologists recognizes that current knowledge of human behavior, population pressures and changes in medical technology challenge the position traditionally held regarding interruption of pregnancy.
>
> We are aware of our nursing role in relation to cooperating with team members in meeting the health care needs of the woman seeking an abortion or sterilization. Genuine concern and compassion for this woman is strongly urged. However, there may

be concern regarding nursing practice and participation in this particular area of health care. It is, therefore, our aim to recommend that an individual's rights must be maintained and safeguarded by written policies.

The Association recommends the following principles and guidelines:

1. Nurses have the responsibility to provide nursing care.
2. Nurses have the right to refuse to assist in the performance of abortions and/or sterilization procedures in keeping with their moral, ethical and/or religious beliefs, except in an emergency when a patient's life is clearly endangered, in which case the questioned moral issue should be disregarded. This refusal should not jeopardize the nurses' employment nor should they be subjected to harrassment or embarrassment because of their refusal.
3. Nurses, in dealing with such patients, should not impose their views on the patients or personnel.
4. Nurses have the right to expect their employers to describe to them the hospital's policies and practices regarding abortions and sterilizations.
5. Nurses have the obligation to inform their employers of their attitudes and beliefs regarding abortions and sterilizations.

Item 2 paves the way for a nurse to make her ethical decision in keeping with her own socioreligious beliefs. In keeping with the democratic ideal it safeguards the beliefs of the nurse by providing that no official or nonofficial action shall be taken against her for exercising her right to act in accordance with her own set of ethics in cases of moral conflict.

While protecting the right of the nurse to hold and practice her own ethical standards the statement also protects the rights of patients who may hold contrary ethical positions. The patient also may not be subjected to abuse or harrassment by staff. This mutual respect for conflicting views about ethics is necessary for the protection of all members of the society.

Along with the new morality there has also emerged a modification of established ethical patterns. Occasionally it is difficult for scientifically trained professionals to understand that many of the seemingly absolute laws of ethics and morality that they hold are really only opinions. It is only as nurses, who by training are often empiricists, come to this realization that they can function more efficiently in our pluralistic society. The variants in ethics as seen through the eyes of the beholder, whether patient, physician, administrator, or nurse, must always be maintained and respected.

**REFERENCES**

1. Means, R. L.: *The Ethical Imperative.* New York, Doubleday & Co., 1970
2. Fletcher, J.: *Situation Ethics: The New Morality.* Philadelphia, Westminster Press, 1966

# The Patient-Client as a Consumer:

## Some Observations on the Changing Professional-Client Relationship

### by Leo G. Reeder

One of the most significant changes that has occurred in the developed societies has been a shift in medical care from curative to preventive types of services. In a system dominated by curative or emergency care there is a "seller's market." The customer is suspect; client-professional relationships tend to be characterized by the traditional mode of interaction so well described in the literature. On the other hand, when prevention of illness is emphasized, the client has to be persuaded that he has a need for medical services such as periodic check-ups. The person has to be encouraged to come into the physician's

**Leo G. Reeder, Ph.D.,** is professor of sociology and professor of public health at the University of California at Los Angeles. He is a co-editor of the recently published second edition of Handbook of Medical Sociology, co-author of Perceptions of Medical Care and is co-editor with E. Gartly Jaco of a new series on Health as a Social Problem.

Condensed from the *Journal of Health & Social Behavior* (December 1972) Vol. 13, pp. 406-412 © 1972 by the American Sociological Association.

office for medical care. Under these circumstances, there are elements of a "buyer's market"; in such situations there is more tendency for the "customers to be right."

A second feature of societal change concerns the growing sophistication with bureaucracy. In the health care field there has been a considerable development of prepaid health care programs organized by private practitioners and others. This development will undoubtedly be accelerated by the federally-encouraged Health Maintenance Organizations. Thus, increasingly, non-welfare, paying patients will receive medical care in some type of organizational milieu. The bureaucratic features of the profession of medicine plus the increasing bureaucratization of delivery of personal health services combine to create institutionalized, more or less standardized, environments that provide standard patterns of experience, attitudes, and values to the participants in the system, providers and consumers alike.

The third feature of societal change to be noted is the development of consumerism. During the decade of the sixties a new concept came into prominence in the delivery of health services in this country. This was the concept of the person as a *consumer* rather than as a patient. Concurrently, the greater focus on the problems of *delivery* of medical services has resulted in increasing use of such terms as "health providers" to replace the more traditional terminology of "doctor." Thus, increasingly we speak of the relationship between health *providers* and *consumers* rather than the doctor-patient relationship. Indeed, it is now generally recognized that we are in the early stages of the "age of the consumer." On a variety of fronts the voice of the consumer is making itself heard in a powerful way: for example, Ralph Nader is a symbol of the consumer movement; the executive branch of government has the President's Committee on Consumer Interests; in Philadelphia and in San Mateo, prisoners have brought suit over failure to provide adequate medical or rehabilitative care; and in the health field the consumer movement received particular impetus through the OEO-sponsored Neighborhood Health Centers. Indeed, the trend toward citizen control of Neighborhood Health Centers is well advanced and sometimes encouraged by officialdom. This trend toward greater consumer involvement in health affairs is prevalent in a variety of contexts. For example, the following declaration was made at a national conference on rehabilitation:

> The consumer must be a vital and fundamental part of the rehabilitation system — or the system is irrelevant

delivering community health services on the basis of continuous consultation with both the producers and the consumers of those services . . . the kinds of community health problems which are emerging and becoming dominant are less amenable to technological solutions and more and more require consumer cooperation and collaboration.

The experiences of Neighborhood Health Centers may be illustrated by comments of Martin Cherkasky in reference to the South Bronx Neighborhood Medical Care Demonstration:

> The providers of medical care no longer have the sole prerogative for decision-making and this is all to the good. Health planners cannot understand groups . . . different from their most intimate collaborative planning and management of these joint health care enterprises.

A recent statement issued by a group of faculty in Schools of Public Health takes note of the trend by calling for the overall mission of Schools for Public Health to include:

> . . . the facilitation of the development of innovative ways of organizing and delivering community health services on the basis of continuous consultation with both the producers and the consumers of those services . . . the kinds of community health problems which are emerging and becoming dominant are less amenable to technological solutions and more and more require consumer cooperation and collaboration.

The mere use of the term "consumers" to replace "clients" initiates a different perspective. As a client, on the one hand, the individual delivers himself into the hands of the professional — who presumably is the sole decision-maker regarding the nature of the services to be delivered. On the other hand, when the individual is viewed as a consumer, he is a purchaser of services and tends to be guided by *caveat emptor*. Thus, the switching of labels tends to change the fabric of the social relationships between practitioners in the health delivery system and their clients.

In patient-practitioner relationships power is lodged in the physician and negotiations and bargainings typically do not occur on an equal basis.

In consumer-provider relationships, *caveat emptor* implies that the consumer has considerably more bargaining power than formerly. He may, under certain circumstances of a changing social structure of the health system, be able to shop in the market place of health care. With the structural relationships undergoing a process of alteration, the behavior of both the professionals and their clientele will be altered.

From another conceptual perspective, consumerism tends to take on some of the characteristics of a social movement — an effort by a large number of people to solve collectively a problem that they feel they have in common. According to this view, the success of social movements depends on the size, organization, and quality of leadership and more upon the extent to which the movement successfully expresses the feelings, resentments, wor-

ries, and concerns of large numbers of people and the "degree to which these movements can be viewed as vehicles for the solution of wide-spread problems." Thus, consumerism in health care may be viewed in terms of *shared perspectives,* i.e., as noted earlier, people in similar situations tend to view their problems alike and to evaluate them similarly. It is in this sense that consumerism may take on some of the aspects of a social movement.

Public statements by health officials and leaders of consumer organizations provide further evidence for viewing consumerism from a social movement perspective. The most outstanding example of this phenomenon is probably the experience of the Office of Economic Opportunity's program of maximum feasible participation by citizens in consumer action programs, particularly in the Neighborhood Health Center's established by OEO. From participation there has emerged a distinct trend toward *control* of such action programs. Eventually, there will be demands for consumer representation on the governing councils of organizations within which the professional and client interact. We can expect that in the medical care field the pressures will continue to build toward consumer representation on hospital boards, prepaid medical care plans, etc.

In addition to consumer representation on governing boards of agencies and institutions delivering professional services, another development may be the employment of an ombudsman.

Increasingly, there is greater recognition given to such an office in service-related organizations such as universities, government, and similar enterprises. It is reasonable to expect that the consumer movement will accelerate the adoption of the ombudsman format to mediate differences between professionals and client-consumers.

As the rules regarding interaction within the organizational or bureaucratic context change, the right to rule on what are legitimate patterns may shift toward the consumer and away from the professional. Thus, the role-set in the interactive system of an organizational setting, as it relates to professional-client relations and possibly to the organizational division of labor, will tend to change.

Of course, it must be recognized that these changing relationships between the professional practitioner and the client-consumer may vary according to such features as: type of practice, type of physician, type of illness, etc. Furthermore, there are at least two varieties of consumer participation that should be explicitly distinguished:

(1) in the arena of health planning and the organization of health services, and

(2) in the regimen of health care itself, e.g., getting medical checkups, smoking cessation, and other preventive health behaviors that require the clients' energies and participation for self-help.

In the former, the processes of change in the professional-client relationship are well-advanced and will undoubtedly continue and perhaps accelerate. In the latter, there may be certain more-or-less enduring features of the traditional model doctor-patient relationship which will set limits on consumer participation.

As the groups representing "consumers" and the groups representing the health professions confront one another, the interactional processes provide a focus for further study. Attention needs to be given to the forms, content, and symbols used in this interactional process. Out of such observations we can gain better understanding of the underlying processes involved in the changing professional-client relationship.

*" . . .it is not enough that we do*
*a technically competent job*
*of healing the patient's body;*
*we must do an equally competent job*
*of safeguarding his dignity and self-esteem.*
*In proportion as we fail in this latter task,*
*we destroy the practical value of our*
*technical competence for the sick person."*

# Illness and Indignity

## Thomas S. Szasz

All of us in the health professions share certain fundamental aspirations and goals, among which the most important are keeping the healthy person healthy; restoring the sick person to health; and, most generally, safeguarding and prolonging life. That these ends are so overwhelmingly good and noble is what makes their pursuit so gratifying, and those in the health professions so richly honored and rewarded.

Life would be simpler than it is if health and longevity were its principal purposes; or if there were no values that often conflict with their pursuit. One of the values that we cherish, and that often conflicts with the pursuit of health at any cost, is dignity.

Dignity is that ineffable yet obvious quality of human encounters that enriches the participants' self-esteem. The process of dignification is characteristically reciprocal; dignified conduct in one person generates dignified conduct in another, and vice versa.

Conversely, indignity is that equally obvious, but much more easily definable quality of human encounters that impoverishes the participants' self-esteem. One of its most common and most tragic forms is the

**Thomas S. Szasz, M.D.** is professor of psychiatry, State University of New York, Upstate Medical Center, Syracuse, New York.

Condensed and reprinted with permission from the *Journal of The American Medical Association*, Volume 227, Number 5, (February 4, 1974), pp. 543–545. Read in part as the commencement address before the College of Health Related Professions, State University of New York, Upstate Medical Center, Syracuse, New York, June 3, 1973.

49

indignity of disability, illness, and old age. Many sick persons behave, simply because of their illness, in ways that make their conduct undignified. When a person loses control over his basic bodily functions, when he cannot work, then—often against his most intense efforts—he is rendered undignified. Language, still the most reliable guide to a people's true sentiments, starkly reveals this intimate connection between illness and indignity. In English, we use the same word to describe an expired passport, an indefensible argument, an illegitimate legal document, and a person disabled by disease. We call each of them "invalid." To be an invalid, then, is to be an invalidated person, a human being stamped "not valid" by the hand of popular opinion. While invalidism carries with it the heaviest burden of indignity, some of this stigma adheres to virtually all illness.

This fact generates two very important problems for persons in the health professions: one is that the sick person's undignified behavior may stimulate the professional's inclination to respond with undignified behavior of his own; the other is that patients disabled in ways that render them grossly undignified may prefer death with dignity to life without it. Let me offer a few observations of each of these.

## The Indignity of Being a Patient

The connections between illness and indignity are, in the main, quite obvious. Because the patient cannot work, cannot take care of himself, and for many other equally good reasons, he perceives himself as suffering not only an illness but also a loss of dignity. Moreover, the patient's loss of dignity often generates a reciprocal loss of respect for him by those around him, especially by his family and physicians. This unfortunate process of degradation is often concealed, though in my opinion never very successfully, by the imagery and vocabulary of paternalism—family and physician treating the patient as if he were a child (or child-like), and the patient treating them as if they were his parents (or superiors).

This fundamental tendency—to "infantilize" the sick person and to "parentify" the healer—manifests itself in countless ways in the everyday practice of medicine. For example, the patient is expected to trust his physician, but the physician need not trust his patient; the patient is expected to impart his intimate bodily and personal experiences to the physician, while the physician may withhold vital information from the patient.

The patient's undignified position vis-a-vis medical authorities is symbolized by the linguistic structure of the medical situation. The patient communicates in ordinary language, which he shares with his physician; the physician communicates partly in the same language, insofar as he speaks *to* his patient, and partly in another language, insofar as he speaks *about* him. The physician's second language is the technical jargon of medicine. The upshot is that patients often do not know or understand what is wrong with them, what is in their medical records, or what drugs they are taking. To be sure, like children or other fearful, humiliated, or oppressed persons, patients often do not want to know these things. Yet even if this were so it would not, in my opinion, justify withholding such information from them. After all, many people do not want to know what is under the hood of an automobile, but we would not accept this as justifying automobile manufacturers in maintaining a systematic policy of withholding this information from car buyers or releasing it to them only under special circumstances.

My point is that many people today accept it as right and proper that patients should not understand their prescriptions or that they should not know what is in their hospital records; at the same time, they object to the indignities which the medical situation often imposes on them. The result of this inarticulated conflict is that people often feel anxious and humiliated at the prospect of seeking medical care and frequently avoid or reject such care altogether.

We must keep in mind that people want and need not only health but also dignity, that often they can obtain health only at the cost of dignity, and that sometimes they prefer not to pay this price. It is obvious, for example, that patients participate most eagerly and most intelligently in medical situations that entail little or no humiliation on their part, and most reluctantly or not at all in those medical situations that entail a great deal of humiliation.

There is a practical lesson in this for all of us: namely, that it is not enough that we do a technically competent job of healing the patient's body; we must do an equally competent job of safeguarding his dignity and self-esteem. In proportion as we fail in this latter task, we destroy the practical value of our technical competence for the sick person.

## Is Health Worth the Price of Dignity?

The irreconcilable conflict that may arise between prolonging life and maintaining dignity was, as were all the fundamental conflicts characteristic of the human condition, well appreciated and articulated by the ancient Greeks. In the "Phaedo," Plato illustrates this dilemma and Socrates' method of resolving it.

The "Death Scene" opens with Socrates and some of his closest friends gathered in anticipation of Socrates drinking the hemlock. After some conversation between Socrates and his friends, Socrates says farewell and asks the executioner to bring the poisoned cup. But Crito urges Socrates to wait, to prolong his life for as long as he may: "But Socrates," he pleads, "I know that other men take the poison quite late, and eat and drink heartily, and even enjoy the company of their chosen friends, after the announcement has been made. So do not hurry; there is still time."

Socrates' reply articulates the distinction between life as a biological process that may and perhaps ought to be prolonged for as long as possible, and as a spiritual pilgrimage that can and should be traversed and ended in a proper manner. This is what Socrates says:

*And those whom you speak of, Crito, naturally do so; for they think that they will be the gainers by so doing. And I naturally shall not do so; for I think that I should gain nothing by drinking the poison a little later but my own contempt for so greedily saving up a life which is already spent.*

The distinction between the death of the body and the end of life, which is the difference between Crito's and Socrates' outlook on life and death, continues to baffle us in the health sciences. The main reason why this is the case is, remarkably, also explained by Socrates.

Crito asks his friend how he wants to be buried. Socrates replies:

*Crito thinks that I am the body which he will presently see as a corpse, and he asks me how he is to bury me. All the arguments which I have used to prove that I shall not remain with you*

*after I have drunk the poison . . . have been thrown away on him. . . . For, dear Crito, you must know that to use words wrongly is not only a fault in itself, it also corrupts the soul. You must be of good cheer, and say that you are burying my body; and you may bury it as you please, and you think right.*

The distinction Socrates makes here between himself and his body is at once obvious and elusive; you know as well as I how often scientifically informed and enlightened people fail to make this distinction.

The richness of "The Death Scene" for our theme is by no means exhausted by my foregoing remarks. There is significance, too, in Socrates' parting words. "Crito," he says, "I owe a cock to Asclepius; do not forget it."

The ritual sacrifice Socrates here requests his friend to make on his behalf refers to the custom of offering, on recovering from sickness, a cock to Asclepius, the god of healing. In other words, Socrates viewed his death as a recovery from an illness, presaging the Christian view of it.

In short, the message I want to bring you is simply this: Do your utmost to exercise your skills in healing, but do not do so by sacrificing dignity, either your patient's or your own—these two being tied together by bonds not unlike those of matrimony, except, especially in these days, stronger. For, if I may paraphrase the Scriptures, what does it profit a man if he gains his health but loses his dignity?

"There is a pervasive belief that the modern nurse is still tied to her nineteenth century stereotype, that the physician is the natural leader of the health team, and that nursing work is for the tender, sympathetic and softhearted, therefore, female."

"We can change things for ourselves instead of being constantly on the changed end of the process. This will require a tenacious grasp of the situations we wish changed and affirmative action in which nurses themselves are the implementers and directors."

# *Freedom for Our Sisters, Freedom for Nursing*

## *Karen T. Lamb*

**Karen Thompson Lamb, R.N., M.A.,** is in the Department of Sociology at the University of Arizona, where she is a candidate for the Ph.D. degree.

Adapted from a paper presented by the author at a joint workshop sponsored by the University of Arizona and Arizona State University in 1973.

Nursing cannot take its rightful place among the professions until the status of women in this society is improved. It is the thesis of this article that nursing and the Women's Rights Movement are inextricably bound together. It is impossible for nursing to achieve real professionalization and lower the drastic drop-out rate among our practitioners, or for us to assume control over ourselves as individuals and as a collectivity, to take more active roles as innovators and instigators of social change, and to develop a career-orientation until we have elevated the position of all women—and of nurses.

Let us look briefly at where women are in the professions, where I think we are in nursing, and at the problems women face that make our road toward professionalization in nursing difficult.

When we look at women's roles in this society we should be appalled at the waste of this country's human resources. Professional fields are just beginning to open up to women, and this only after decades of struggle. Women in the professions are sorely under-represented, and are generally found doing the child care, nurturance, and housekeeping of the professions. Rarely are women, who make up the bulk of the teaching profession, found administering and managing their own profession. And in medicine, where women make up 7.8 percent of the total number of physicians, the most popular specialty for women is pediatrics, the least popular, surgery. The notion that women have high manual dexterity, and therefore are better than males at the monotonous job of putting in ball bearings in electronic plants does not seem to extend to working in the brain or abdomen in the surgical theater.

Salary-wise, there is still a $4,000 a year income differential between the full-time working man and the full-time working woman. At a symposium on women in the scientific professions held recently at the Massachusetts Institute of Technology, a panelist stated that this country has proceeded on the theory that one does not really expect any significant contribution from women.

Nursing has its own peculiar problems, not the least of which is that it is called a "woman's profession." The term "profession" should be sufficient if, indeed, nursing is a profession. To continue to combine such terms as woman doctor, woman lawyer, and male nurse smacks of sexism. Why is there a need to specify if we are not pointing out a deviant from the norm?

It is difficult for many to hold the opinion that nursing is a profession when we review the criteria for a profession as outlined by Flexner, Merton, and Bixler: extended periods of learning in institutions of higher education, systems of honorary and monetary rewards, ethics formalized into codes, and autonomy. More important than whether we consider ourselves professionals, this society does not. There is a pervasive belief that the modern nurse is still tied to her nineteenth century stereotype, that the physician is the natural leader of the health team, and that nursing work is for the tender, sympathetic and soft-hearted, therefore, female. The fantasy of medicine, and the idealization of the physician's grand assault on disease, also casts nurses as entirely dependent on the perception and orders of this great healer. And since the practice of medicine, dentistry, and pharmacy is viewed as masculine and nursing as feminine, the result is sex segregation. Like other forms of segregation, sex segregation results in communication, social, and psychological barriers.

In 1948, anthropologist R. L. Birdwhistell reported views of the nurse of people from three social classes. These views are quoted here because the image of our practitioners has not changed in the past twenty-five years.

According to lower-income groups,

> . . . nursing is one of the noblest of all professions. The nurse is one who has bettered herself by education and who in her everyday life is surrounded by excitement, glamour, and interesting people. . . . (She is) in a position in which she will be able to make a good marriage and to give her husband and children the advantages of her acquired knowledge.

There were no particular comments concerning the nurse's morality by the women other than that the girls were "well chaperoned during training." The males agreed with the fact that the girls were "looked after" by the head nurses, but added with sly snickers that the doctors probably "had a lot of fun with them". . . . This group viewed the nurse as a technical expert. She takes temperatures, gives hypodermics, and writes knowingly on report pads. By the members of this group the nurse was rated very high as a professional—"almost a doctor!"

To the middle-class respondents, the nurse is a semi-skilled to skilled individual who is variedly regarded by the women as someone who is working a while before marriage, who is widowed, divorced, or who is a "career woman" (which is the middle-class woman's description of a woman who can't get a husband or who is a neglectful wife). . . . The women distrust the nurse and regard her as a husband hunter capable of employing unfair tactics. (Incidentally, the nurse is not alone in this; the middle-class woman tends to regard her husband as easy prey for any designing woman who can get him alone.). . . . The men of this group talked of nurses as "easy marks." Yet they seemed to have respect for them, considering a nurse to be a "good fellow" with considerable knowledge which in a crisis could be useful. Several of the men in this group were married to nurses. These stressed the fact that their wives were "different" and that they had married the nurses when they were young. Both males and females were somewhat ambivalent in their attitude toward nurses.

Upper-income respondents viewed the nurse as a skilled menial, somewhat higher in social prestige than the manicurist or hairdresser, but considerably below the social worker. . . . Her job is viewed as an unpleasant one. She was regarded as "nice" to males and cruel to women, particularly those in childbirth. . . . The nurse was not regarded by these upper-class women as a threat. . . . Both males and females assumed that there would be casual affairs between the nurse and her male patients, but reiterated, "It couldn't come to anything" (meaning marriage).

If there is any validity to these images of the nurse, and we find them offensive, then two or three choices seem open to us. First, we can let men outside the profession change things for us — if and when they are so inclined. But we may have a long wait. Choice two: We can invite and encourage men to come into the profession, and promote them rapidly to the top over equally or better qualified women in the hope that they will not stand for the situation as it is and will better our profession for us. Choice three: We can change things for ourselves instead of being constantly on the changed-end of the process. This will require a tenacious grasp of the situations we wish changed and affirmative action in which nurses themselves are the implementers and directors.

## AFFIRMATIVE ACTION IN NURSING

What kinds of action might be taken to bring women and nursing out of second-class citizenship? We cannot become a true profession unless the society in which we work perceives us as a profession, until our practitioners internalize the attitudes of professionals, and until we behave as professionals. Our first step should be to examine the behavior of our practitioners and our profession both when we are together in the educational and work situation and when we interact with society. Our goal is to bring nursing as a profession, and nurses as women and practitioners, into the mainstream of this society. We are not asking for a radically restructured society. We are asking for reform, not revolution. We realize that in seeking reform we must be willing to take more responsibility than we have done in the past. That will be our part of the bargain: assumption of more responsibility in exchange for the rewards that will accrue to us as individual women and as a true profession.

*Individual Behavior* — Here the goal is to encourage women to view nursing as a career. But developing curriculum further in the direction of science or toward preparing practitioners to become mini-physicians is not the direction we need to take. We should be concerned with the *quality* of the woman who wishes to become a nurse. We need to know what *nursing* is for this candidate. Figures available in the late 1960s show that only 65.3 percent of licensed nurses were practicing nursing. The basic questions to be asked are: What did the inactive 31.4 percent want to contribute to nursing in the first place? How much time and talent were they willing to expend? For how long? What did they hope to gain from their profession? Is it possible that the majority of women who enter our schools and colleges have not the faintest idea of becoming career and professional women?

We must work to eradicate the notion that we are preparing other than the full professional. We must start to change notions about women's careers at the moment candidates to schools of nursing present themselves at the school door. We must work to end the attitude that interruptions in a woman's pursuit of her career can and will be tolerated. Our practitioners must insist that husbands share the responsibility of the home. We cannot continue to support the idea that a woman should look for a career that *she* can manage along with her family responsibilities.

Educating practitioners is costly in time, money, and resources. We must commit ourselves to educating practitioners for a life-time career, not an interrupted, intermittent, half-hearted and uncommitted practice of nursing. It is perfectly proper, in my opinion, to set up counseling and orientation sessions for candidates applying to nursing schools in which potential nurses are told they are embarking on a professional career. School administrators and educators must get across to students that they are mature adults, and as mature adults, are *automatically* assumed to have made arrangements for the management of their families, spouses, and mates before committing themselves to a nursing program.

Moreover, until such a time as occupational counseling is desexed, nursing must take responsibility for this area as well. Considering the few opportunities traditionally open to women, in that initial counseling session we must, if we have integrity, encourage women to examine other careers as well as nursing. Public high school vocational and professional counseling for women continues to shuttle women into secretarial schools, nursing, and teaching. It certainly is realistic to question how many of those hundreds of thousands of drop-out nurses are the result of misguided vocational counseling, boredom, lack of challenge, or how many represent frustrated doctors, lawyers, writers, or researchers. It is probably less costly to nursing to have a high drop-out rate in the initial counseling sessions and to be more certain of the quality and commitment of those who do become practitioners.

*Interaction with the Community* – Nursing must encourage stronger community involvement as an integral part of curriculum. Nursing must not prepare *only* the bedside practitioner who administers one-to-one care, but we must expand our knowledge and practice within the community. Both graduate and student nurses have more knowledge that should be utilized in the decision-making process than the majority of persons who now occupy positions in community agencies and on governmental boards and commissions. Involvement must begin as a part of the basic course of study.

Traditionally, women have been denied decision-making positions. We must work to place women in these positions. That can be done in at least two ways. One, recruit women into nursing who will share with us knowledge gained from other roles and positions they have occupied in the community. If an applicant cannot envision herself as developing other roles in addition to bedside nurse, then perhaps she would be more comfortable in less exacting occupations.

The second approach is to develop additional roles within the community, such as internships under community health administrators, and appointments to boards, commissions, and citizens advisory groups involved with health issues. Urban planning and air pollution advisory boards, health, welfare, and hospital service boards, consumer commissions, parks and recreation, planning and zoning, budget and finance commissions are just a few of the roles that have direct implications for the health of the community. Internships can be arranged on hospital boards and health facilities, and nursing students can be encouraged to intern in local and state legislative bodies for an even more encompassing perspective of community life. This type of program could legitimately be called "clinical practice on the community and state level." Career-oriented persons such as physicians and attorneys do not stick to "doctoring" or "lawyering," for days that begin at 7 a.m. and end at 3 p.m. These professionals are involved in community life in varied ways and roles. So, too, must nurses develop their citizen roles in addition to developing nursing knowledge.

*Interaction with Government or Society* — We must encourage nurses to write and introduce legislation at all levels of government and within our organizations. Women must run for elected office. Otherwise, we cannot end the double standard which ensures that women are never the directors of programs.

We can begin within our own groups inside and outside of nursing to support women's candidacies for elected, appointed, and salaried positions. It should be reiterated that the major decisions which affect us as a profession are made from outside and include the medical profession and government, both predominantly male. It is not discriminatory to support women in preference to men, given comparable credentials, until women have equal access to *all* top-level decision-making positions. There is no shortage of qualified women; it is the positions that are in short supply, and it seems that women's support and encouragement of each other may also be in limited supply.

Part of our battle will be won by the use of legal tools—several of which are available for use now. Others, such as the Equal Rights Amendment (ERA), are on the way.

Inside our walls, we should use the most powerful legal tools we have, including the powers invested in the Office of Federal Contract Compliance (OFCC) and the Equal Employment Opportunity Commission (EEOC). The OFCC is empowered to withhold federal funds from any institution if that institution is found not to be in compliance with the law. The principle here is simple—our government states that institutions are not allowed to use federal funds to perpetuate discrimination against the very citizens who pay the taxes. The Equal Employment Opportunity Commission stands ready to handle violations in employment as outlined under the Civil Rights Act of 1964. Many women have not realized that they have worked their entire lives in employment situations that are in direct violation of their legal rights. It is nursing's responsibility to inform its practitioners of their civil rights and work with them to achieve full civil citizenship.

In addition to legal weapons, each of us has several small- and middle-range theories which we frequently use for our patients' benefit but which may also be used to change others' behavior toward us. Theories of ecology and spatial arrangements, small group theory, and group dynamics can easily be applied in hospitals, and should help to break down barriers to communication among health-team members. Reward and punishment theory, learning theory, and stimulus-response theory also seem to be effective theories for modifying behavior. We must consider carefully the behaviors we are now rewarding and the implications these behaviors hold for the status of women.

## CONCLUSION

Certainly many nurses have taken the responsibilities of full citizenship throughout our history, frequently without the rewards. Many of us are proud that nursing has traditionally been close to the most critical issues that have faced our society. Certainly we care for the end products of an over-populated and environmentally contaminated world. Certainly we have been close to poverty and misery. Certainly we are close to the major demands of the Women's Rights Movement and much of the leadership of this movement comes from nurses. Many of us personally know the problems of obtaining safe child care, and we know intimately exclusion from institutions of higher education.

Who says women can't work together, that we are non-innovative, lack creativity, and are not prepared to be social changers? If we do not expect to succeed, if we retreat in the face of opposition, if we continue to "pretend" that we are dealing with matters of critical importance, then we set in motion a chain of behaviors that may lead to division and conquest. We have only to look around us at the achievements of women. We are learning that sisterhood is indeed powerful—for ourselves and for other women.

". . . full utilization of
true nursing skills
can be realized
only if professional nurses
attend only to
clinical activities. . . ."

# ON THE HORIZON: THE ALL-R.N. NURSING STAFF

*Luther Christman*

**Luther Christman, Ph.D.** is dean of the College of Nursing and Allied Health Sciences and vice president of Nursing Affairs at Rush University, Chicago, Illinois.

**"This thing** we've called team nursing all these years is going to have to go. It can't function. It only produces mediocrity in the delivery of health care," says Luther Christman, R.N., Ph.D., Professor and Dean of Nursing at Rush University's College of Nursing and Allied Health Sciences in Chicago and Vice-President for Nursing Affairs at Rush-Presbyterian-St. Luke's Medical Center.

"No matter how elegant the nursing plan was in its conception," Dr. Christman insists, "it loses all of its elegance as soon as someone other than a competent registered nurse delivers the care. Everyone said we had to have team nursing because of the nursing shortage. But there was a nursing shortage only because we had team nursing. With this system, everyone is busy *watching* patient care instead of *giving* it."

According to Dr. Christman, "An all-RN nursing staff is the necessity of the future if we are to deliver to patients the quality of care that is now possible." He contends, however, that full utilization of true nursing skills can be realized only if professional nurses attend only to clinical activities — those acts which assist in preventing, arresting, or reversing pathological states. Accordingly, if all nonclinical activities — those of a hotel-housekeeping nature — were assigned to a general purpose worker, ". . . the patient would soon learn to depend on this person to fill these needs, and on the nurse for his clinical needs."

"This general purpose worker would experience more work satisfaction than hospital aides now get from the dull, uncertain, routine and repetitive tasks that comprise their day. Furthermore, accountability for care could be fixed with more certainty."

Dr. Christman's aim is more efficient, more effective nursing care.

". . . it has been demonstrated that an all-R.N. staff is not only feasible but that it can greatly increase quality and decrease cost of patient care."

He points out that in studies conducted at the University of Michigan and at Vanderbilt University, it has been demonstrated that an all-RN staff is not only feasible but that it can greatly increase quality and decrease cost of patient care.

"The most costly worker in the nursing department is not the nurse with a master's degree, but the nurse's aide. Why? An activity analysis showed that although aides' hourly rates were less than RN's, aides had 20% more down time than RN s."

If Dr. Christman's proposal sounds idealistic, he is at least practicing what he preaches. At Rush-Presbyterian-St. Luke's Medical Center, each aide who leaves is replaced by a registered nurse. At present, there is an entire reorganization of care being implemented at Rush by nurses, physicians, and persons in hospital administration to synchronize their joint efforts around the patients.

By making the RN's role entirely clinical, Dr. Christman hopes to promote professionalism among nurses and pave the way toward a working interdependence between nurses, physicians, and administrators. At Rush, where equality and interdependence between doctors and nurses is becoming the rule instead of the exception, RNs have been appointed to the medical faculty. But Dr. Christman stresses that they're there because they've met certain competency requirements. "Competency is the key," he says. "Nurses can't just say, 'I'm a nurse so I'm entitled to equality.'"

Having first achieved his national reputation as a clinician — not as an educator — Dr. Christman has long championed clinical leadership in the profession. He served on the first national committee established to develop the nurse specialist and chaired the first national conference to try to pave the way for this role.

Congruent with his clinical orientation, Dr. Christman makes the following proposal: "A few medical centers need to develop very outstanding clinical nursing care programs. This development must be accompanied by imaginative clinical research and high quality clinical education. Out of this total development will evolve centers of excellence in nursing. In this way, the nursing care of patients can be improved immensely."

Condensed with permission of the National Association of Social Workers, from *Social Work*, Volume 18, Number 4, (July, 1973), pp. 10–18.

# *Wyatt* v. *Stickney:* rights of the committed

## *Charles S. Prigmore and Paul R. Davis*

It is not always realized that judges have the power to make policy decisions not only on the strength of their own individual values but on that of changing public values as well. But now the potentially important role of judges in extending individual rights to clients of social services is beginning to emerge, making possible a radical transformation of the social services as we have known them.

Many court decisions on the right of institutionalized mental patients to adequate treatment have been made since 1960. In one notable case, *Rouse v. Cameron,* it was acknowledged that there might be a constitutional right to treatment, but no guidelines were promulgated. This right was not fully and conclusively applied until 1971-1972, when the orders and decrees known as *Wyatt v. Stickney* were given in U.S. Middle District Court of Alabama. The story of this landmark case is told in this article.

## THE BACKGROUND

Bryce State Hospital is a custodial institution accommodating about 5,000 mental patients. It is an agriculture-oriented facility that has been expected to pay much of its own way. Legislative appropriations have been meager and the staff has been largely untrained and poorly paid. The physician-to-patient ratio has been in the order of 250 to 1 and patient stay excessively long. Little con-

**Charles S. Prigmore, Ph.D.,** is professor, School of Social Work, University of Alabama.

**Paul R. Davis** is editor, Selma Times-Journal, Selma, Alabama. At the time this article was written, he was a member of the Human Rights Committee, Partlow State School and Hospital.

tact was maintained with the patient's home community. Until six years ago, it was rigidly segregated; black patients were hidden away at a century-old army outpost near Mobile.

Another institution, Partlow State School and Hospital, housed approximately 2,500 retardates. Its physical appearance, program, and staff-to-patient ratio have been similar to those of Bryce Hospital. Its program and policies have been confused and divided, chiefly because of a lack of agreement as to whether it should be a medical or educational facility. As many as 500 of its residents worked without pay on the institution's farm. Partlow too was segregated, with blacks in the worst of the antiquated buildings.

In October 1970 the Alabama Board of Mental Health and a new commissioner of mental health, Dr. Stonewall B. Stickney, released over 100 employees because of budgetary considerations. Ninety-nine of these employees instituted court action, claiming they were terminated without cause, without notice, and without a hearing. It was further alleged in the action that patients would be deprived of proper treatment because of the terminations. U.S. District Judge Frank Johnson expressed interest in the patients' claim that they were not receiving adequate treatment (the employees' suit was dismissed because technically it did not raise a constitutional question). The action at this point became *Wyatt v. Stickney,* Ricky Wyatt being a patient of Bryce Hospital. The suit was filed as a class action on behalf of all patients at Bryce Hospital, and the judge later granted plaintiffs' motion to add to the lawsuit patients confined at Searcy Hospital, formerly the all-black state hospital for the mentally ill—and residents at Partlow State Hospital.

Dr. Stickney is a psychiatrist with a strong orientation toward community treatment and a particular interest in prevention of institutionalization through mental health services in the schools. His original intention in terminating the employees at Bryce was to divert funds to the emerging comprehensive community mental health centers throughout the state and to deemphasize traditional hospital services. He became a willing adversary in the action brought by the patients, since his aim like theirs was to create a more viable system of care and treatment for the mentally ill and retarded in Alabama.

Dr. Stickney's original recommendation of "bulldozer" therapy for the old facilities was approved by professional groups, but not by the state's physician-dominated mental health board. After running into strong opposition, he chose another course. He found a friend in Dr. James Folsom, director of the Tuscaloosa Veterans Administration Hospital. Dr. Folsom was putting into practice at his hospital new programs that were attracting national attention. With reality orientation and attitude therapy, he rapidly reduced his patient population.

Stickney enlisted Folsom to start the new programs in the state hospitals. However, Dr. Folsom encountered a century-old departmental system that he could not change at Bryce, so he turned his attention to the all-black Searcy Hospital near Mobile. The director here was willing to go along with any change that would result in progress at his hospital. Not until the transformation at Searcy was under way was another effort made to apply the new ideas to Bryce.

The going was still rough. Stickney and Folsom came up with a game plan. Money was short; they announced a mass layoff at Bryce. To keep the institution out of the red, the layoffs involved many at the upper end of the pay scale—professionals.

That was the birth of the *Wyatt v. Stickney* lawsuit. The professionals who did not accept the new programs were fired, and in their attempt to regain their jobs, they raised the question about the quality of patient care with a greatly reduced professional staff.

## THE ORIGINAL ORDER

The order in the original *Wyatt v. Stickney* case was given on March 12, 1971. Briefly, Judge Johnson determined that programs of treatment at Bryce State Hospital were scientifically and medically inadequate and deprived patients of their constitutional rights. The court gave state officials six months to promulgate and implement appropriate standards.

The judge observed that the patients were, for the most part, involuntarily committed through noncriminal proceedings without the constitutional protections afforded defendants in criminal proceedings. "When patients are so committed for treatment purposes they unquestionably have a constitutional right to receive such individual treatment as will give each of them a realistic opportunity to be cured or to improve [their] mental condition."[1] Without adequate treatment, the judge regarded the hospital as a penitentiary in which a person could be held indefinitely for no convicted offense. "The purpose of involuntary hospitalization for treatment," he said, must be *treatment* and not mere custodial care or punishment. . . . The failure to provide suitable and adequate treatment to the mentally ill cannot be justified by lack of staff or facilities."[2]

The court ordered the defendants (the commissioner and deputy commissioner of the Department of Mental Health, the members of the Board of Mental Health, the governor, and the probate judge who holds commitment authority to Bryce Hospital) to file within ninety days a precise definition of the mission and function of the hospital, a specific plan for appropriate and adequate treatment, and a report on the implementation of the unit-team approach. The failure to implement fully within six months from the date of the order a treatment program providing an adequate opportunity for each patient to be cured or to improve his or her mental condition would necessitate the court's appointing a panel of experts in mental health to determine what standards would be required.

## BRYCE AND SEARCY

On September 23, 1971, defendants filed their final report, and the court concluded on December 10, 1971, that they had failed to plan and implement a treatment program satisfying minimum medical and constitutional requisites. The program was deficient in three fundamental areas. It failed to provide (1) a humane psychological and physical environment, (2) qualified staff in numbers sufficient to provide adequate treatment, and (3) individualized treatment plans. The court ordered a formal hearing at which the parties and friends of the court could submit proposed standards for constitutionally adequate treatment. At the hearing, authorities on mental health appeared and testified, and supporting briefs were subsequently filed.

The court approved a set of standards but stressed that they were only medical and constitutional minimums and that defendants should provide physical conditions and treatment programs that substantially exceed the approved minimums. The court also appointed committees to review research proposals and rehabilitation programs and to safeguard the dignity and human rights of patients at both Bryce and Searcy. The committees were also instructed to advise and assist patients who alleged that their legal rights were infringed or that the mental health board had failed to comply with court-ordered guidelines.

The court warned that it would not accept lack of operating funds as a justification for failure to comply. In the event of failure of the legislature and the board to meet the need for funds, the court stated that it would be necessary to take affirmative steps, including appointment of a master, to ensure adequate funding.

Defendants were ordered to prepare and file with the court within six months a report detailing the progress on the implementation of the order.

## PARTLOW

Judge Johnson determined that there is no viable distinction between the mentally ill and the mentally retarded regarding their right to appropriate care when they are civilly confined to public mental hospitals. Thus the only constitutional justification for civilly committing a mental retardate is habilitation, and it follows that once such a person is committed, he has an

67

inviolable constitutional right to habilitation.

Judge Johnson applied this right to the Partlow situation by considering whether prevailing conditions there conformed to minimum standards constitutionally required of an institution for mental retardates. It was demonstrated that deplorable provisions for safety and sanitation, understaffed wards, and overcrowding led to serious accidents and even deaths. The judge concluded that conditions were grossly substandard, and the court ordered the establishment of minimum standards for constitutional care and training at Partlow. Again, these standards were described as minimum, only an approach to the ideal that the defendants ought to aim for.

As at Bryce and Searcy, a human rights committee of seven members was established at Partlow. This committee had the same responsibilities as in the other hospitals, and was given in addition the right to inspect the records of the institution and to interview residents and staff.

The operation of Partlow was considered to suffer from an absence of administrative and managerial organization, intensified by the lack of dynamic, permanent leadership. The court ordered the employment within sixty days of a professionally qualified and experienced administrator on a permanent basis. Failure to make such an appointment would result in the designation of a master.

The defendants were ordered to prepare and file with the court in six months a report detailing their progress on the implementation of the order regarding Partlow.

## MINIMUM STANDARDS

The constitutional standards approved by the court include the following rights:

1. Patients have a right to privacy and dignity.

2. Patients have a right to the least restrictive conditions necessary to achieve the purposes of commitment.

3. Patients have the same rights to visitation and telephone communications as patients at other public hospitals.

4. Patients have an unrestricted right to send sealed mail.

5. Patients have a right to be free from unnecessary or excessive medication.

6. Patients have a right to be free from physical restraint and isolation. Except in emergency situations, patients may be physically restrained or placed in isolation only on the order of a qualified mental health professional

7. Patients have a right not to be subjected to experimental research without the express and informed consent of the patient and his guardian or next of kin, after consultation with legal counsel.

8. Patients have a right not to

be subjected to treatment procedures such as lobotomy, electroconvulsive treatment, aversive reinforcement conditioning, or other unusual or hazardous treatment procedures without their express and informed consent after consultation with counsel.

9. Patients have a right to receive prompt and adequate medical treatment for any physical ailments.

10. Patients have a right to wear their own clothes and to keep and use their own personal possessions except insofar as such clothes or possessions may be determined by a qualified mental health professional to be dangerous or otherwise inappropriate.

11. Patients have a right to regular physical exercise several times a week.

12. No patient shall be required to perform labor that involves the operation and maintenance of the hospital or for which the hospital is under contract with an outside organization.

13. A patient has a right to a humane psychological and physical environment within the hospital facilities.

14. The number of patients in a multi-patient room shall not exceed six.

15. There will be one toilet provided for each eight patients and one lavatory for each six patients.

16. There will be one bathtub or shower for each fifteen patients. If a central bathing area is provided, each shower stall must be separated by curtains to ensure privacy.

17. The diet for patients will provide at a minimum the recommended daily dietary allowance as developed by the National Academy of Sciences.

18. For each 250 patients the hospital shall have a minimum of two social workers with the MSW degree and five with the BA degree.

19. Each patient shall have a comprehensive physical and mental examination and review of behavioral status within 48 hours after admission to the hospital.

20. Each patient shall have an individualized treatment plan.

21. Upon the patient's admission, he and his family, guardian, or next of kin shall promptly receive written notice, in language he understands, of all the standards for adequate treatment.

For Partlow, the above standards were applied together with some additional ones, including the following:

1. No mentally retarded person shall be admitted to the institution if services and programs in the community can afford him adequate habilitation.

2. No borderline or mildly retarded person shall be a resident of the institution.

3. Residents shall have a right to receive suitable educational services regardless of chronological age, degree of retardation, or accompanying disabilities or handicaps.

4. As part of his habilitation plan, each resident shall have an individualized post-institutionalization plan.

5. Residents shall lose none of the rights enjoyed by citizens of Alabama and the United States solely by reason of their admission or commitment to the institution, except as determined by an appropriate court.

6. The institution shall provide, under appropriate supervision, suitable opportunities for the resident's interaction with members of the opposite sex.

7. Medication shall not be used as punishment, for the convenience of staff, as a substitute for a habilitation program, or in quantities that interfere with the resident's habilitation program.

8. Corporal punishment shall not be permitted.

9. Residents may voluntarily engage in habilitation labor at nonprogram hours for which the institution would otherwise have to pay an employee, provided the specific labor or any change in labor is (a) an integrated part of the resident's habilitation plan and approved as a habilitation activity by a qualified mental retardation professional responsible for supervising the resident's habilitation; (b) supervised by a staff member to oversee the habilitation aspects of the activity; and (c) compensated in accordance with the minimum wage laws of the U.S. Fair Labor Standards Act.

10. Qualified staff in numbers sufficient to administer adequate habilitation shall be provided, including one social worker for each sixty residents.

11. Each resident discharged to the community shall have a program of transitional habilitation assistance.

## IMPLICATIONS

In *Wyatt v. Stickney,* the court clearly defined the purposes of commitment to public hospitals for the mentally ill and mentally retarded, affirmed the rights of patients or residents to specific services and opportunities once a commitment had been effected, established minimum standards of care and habilitation, established standards of staff qualification and appropriate staff-resident ratios, indicated appropriate approaches to transitional care and postinstitutional care, and determined that institutions for the retarded should be considered educational facilities. Significantly, the court did not concede that lack of funds could be used as a valid reason for not affording the stated minimum standards.

A review of the appellate actions now under way in *Wyatt v. Stickney* indicates that the court's order and decree will probably be upheld in every respect except possibly that of forcing the state legislature to appropriate the funds considered adequate by the court. This issue, however, has been moot since the state Department of Mental Health began to receive federal grants under the Social Security Act.

Federal funds for "transitional" services were largely overlooked for a number of years. This was not so much an oversight as an unwillingness to look for alternatives to institutionalization. Active treatment programs designed to return mentally ill and retarded people to the community had never been seriously considered.

For that matter, most people in the community also believed the mentally ill and retarded should be kept in institutions. Not only the public but members of the mental health board were skeptical about halfway houses, group homes, sheltered workshops, and day-care centers. Those raising most of the questions, and most of the fears, were the medical doctors who through the years had sent hundreds of persons to mental institutions.

If the decision in *Wyatt v. Stickney* becomes the law of the land, mental hospitals and schools for the retarded will hold a decreasing number of people because they will not be permitted to become dumping grounds. They will be closely linked to other community services. They will tend to attract and hold well-qualified staff. The physical facilities will be more nearly adequate. The average stay should be briefer and recommitment less likely to occur. The old stigmas and self-fulfilling prophecies should tend to fade.

A major impact will be to force the rapid development of community-based services. When hospitals and schools for the mentally ill and retarded must, by law, be more nearly adequate, they will obviously become more expensive to operate. The search for alternative programs will be undertaken in earnest, impelled by the desire to save funds.

The central constitutional position established in *Wyatt v. Stickney* is that involuntary commitment requires the granting of a wide range of rights to residents of public hospitals and institutions. However, Judge Johnson stated that "the burden falls squarely upon the institution to prove that a particular resident has not been involuntarily committed, and only if defendants satisfy this difficult burden of proof will the court be confronted with whether the voluntarily committed resident [too] has a right to habilitation." [3] If it turns out that the voluntarily committed resident does have a constitutional right to habilitation, it will probably follow that once a government accepts responsibility for providing a social service, the recipient has a constitutional right to service that is adequate.

### REFERENCES

1. See *Wyatt v. Stickney,* 325 Federal Supplement, p. 784.
2. Ibid.
3. *Wyatt v. Stickney,* 344 Federal Supplement, p. 390.

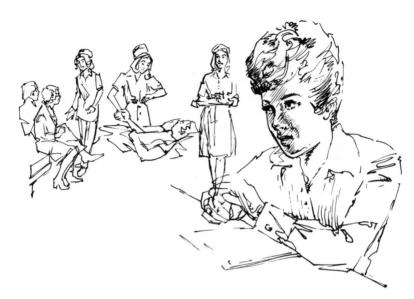

# Nursing Education
## As It Affects
## Specialty Nursing Care

*Jerome P. Lysaught*

**Jerome P. Lysaught, Ed.D.** is professor of Education, College of Education; and professor of Medical Education and Communications, School of Medicine and Dentistry, The University of Rochester, Rochester, New York. He was formerly director of the National Commission for the Study of Nursing and Nursing Education.

Condensed and reprinted with permission from the *Journal of Obstetric, Gynecologic and Neonatal Nursing,* Volume 3, Number 1, (January-February 1974), pp. 17–22. This article is adapted from a presentation by Dr. Lysaught at the 1973 Conference of NAACOG District VII at New Orleans in October. Copyright © 1974 by Harper & Row, Inc.

> *". . . nursing no longer*
> *has a fifty year margin*
> *to mend its educational problems.*
> *Further failure of the profession*
> *to put its educational structure*
> *in tune with the times*
> *is likely to lead to*
> *a disillusionment so great*
> *that nursing's very relevance*
> *will be in doubt."*

For the past six years, I have become more and more skeptical about some aspects of nursing education, particularly its relationship to the real world of practice and patient care. A short statement drawn from the report of Former Secretary Richardson's Committee to study the expanded role of the nurse pinpoints my concern:

> We believe that the future of nursing must encompass a substantially larger place within the community of the health professions. Moreover, we believe that extending the scope of nursing practice is essential if this Nation is to achieve the goal of equal access to health services for all its citizens.

I don't know how anyone could state the issue more bluntly than that. If the practice role of the nurse clinician is to be expanded, however, our educational system and patterns must function in ways compatible with that end.

This is the paradox we face: On the one hand, it is stated that to meet the health care needs of the nation we need more practitioners functioning in expanded nursing roles. On the other, we know that our educational system is not producing such practitioners and is seemingly reluctant to change it ways.

Most of the problems facing nursing education today were described by the Goldmark Commission in 1923. Twenty-five years later Esther Lucile Brown highlighted many of the same problems and recommended appropriate changes. The National Commission, some 50 years later, is laboring to solve many of the same difficulties. But nursing no longer has a 50-year margin to mend its educational problems. Further failure of the profession to put its educational structure in tune with the times is likely to lead to a disillusionment so great that nursing's very relevance will be in doubt.

## Six Fundamental Problems

I suggest that there are six fundamental problems in nursing education that have a particular impact on the practice of all nurses, particularly those who seek to expand and specialize their roles and functions.

### Lack of Single System

The first of the six fundamental problems in nursing education is that it still has not developed a single rational system for preparatory education. Of all the professions, or near-professions, nursing alone enters the last quarter of the twentieth century with a bifurcated, belligerent system half located in the collegiate mainstream and half within the hospital schools of nursing. Year after year this patchwork quilt takes its toll of individual nurses caught between incompatible segments. Each graduate of a hospital school who wishes to continue up the educational ladder finds this at best a hazardous climb, and at worst a damnable hoax.

Goldmark proposed a collegiate system of nursing education 50 years ago; Brown recommended a collegiate system of nursing education 25 years ago; the National Commission has had the satisfaction of seeing, for the first time ever, the majority of institutions and the majority of students under the collegiate roof. It is time to establish a single, rational, compatible system for nursing education that will not frustrate career mobility for the nurse practitioner.

### Two-Year vs Four-Year Programs

The second problem in nursing education is related to the first. If the Commission wants a rational system for nursing education, it also demands that it be an articulated system with proper bridging between two- and the four-year programs. This recommendation, of course, flies in the face of all the nonsense that has ever been generated by nursing educators about the differences between two- and four-year programs. Most nursing curricula are generally alike whether in a two-, three-, or four-year program. In terms of objective results, state licensing board scores, blind studies of beginning practitioners, and other measures, there are at least as many similarities as there are differences among all kinds of educational institutions.

I submit that most of the "differences" are easily explained by simple maturation as by the "inherent and unique qualities" of the baccalaureate program. What is needed are genuine lower and upper division sequences in nursing, and genuine differences between two- and four-year collegiate programs, as well as ready access from the two-year college into the third year of the baccalaureate program.

## Unchallenged Common Beliefs

One of the reasons that the two- and four-year nursing curricula are not more different lies in the third problem of professional education, a common belief held so uncritically that few realize that it has never actually been examined.

Because nursing education grew up in the hospital setting, it was taken for granted that nurses should be trained to work in that environment. But 88 percent of the health care problems in this country have nothing to do with hospital services. Rather, they are problems of health maintenance, disease prevention, primary care, and nonacute illness. This is really a figure to conjure with because, at the present time, approximately 89 percent of all full-time nurse practitioners in this country are in hospital or hospital-related activities.

Worse than this, however is the fact that almost all preparatory programs in nursing are turning out nurses whose clinical instruction is shaped entirely around the episodic environment. What is needed is the development of alternative clinical tracks leading to beginning practitioner skills in *both* episodic and distributive care with individuals permitted to elect their areas of concentration. This would further mean that the present baccalaureate programs will not only have to add genuine upper division sequences but will also have to increase their alternatives and strengthen specialization in clinical nursing roles. It is now time for nurses to insist that nursing education prepare practitioners across the entire range of consumer needs, including the ability to care for the well and the sick.

## Separation of Education and Practice

The reason that nurse educators don't teach expanded role functioning and extended clinical practice is related to the fourth problem in professional education—the separation of education and practice. Most nurse educators are simply not capable of serving in an expert role for the edification of their students. The day we begin to "push" clinical instruction "down" into the lower division, develop true upper division courses in nursing science and practice, and insist that the nurse faculty be able to practice what they preach, we will have solved our problem of separation between education and service.

If nursing is to remain relevant, nurse educators must return to practice and establish themselves as models of excellence. And if nursing is to be truly a full profession, it must be treated as an applied clinical science without a false division between education and practice.

It seems almost ludicrous to point out that teaching and practice are but opposite sides of the same coin in a clinical profession, but nursing education has behaved as if teaching and practice were mutually exclusive.

Nursing service and nursing education must start working together and striving for excellence in clinical teaching and continuing excellence in care provision that will be mutually supportive. This effort should begin at once.

## Lack of Continuing Education

The fifth problem in nursing education is an over concern for preparatory education to the detriment of well planned, continuing clinical education. There is a rising tide of legislation aimed at mandating continuing education for relicensure in nursing. This effort to require continuous leaning has served to highlight how little there is to offer nurses who really are committed to the extension of their clinical skills.

In part, the lack of continuing education in clinical nursing is the result of separation between educators and service people. It is also due to organizational separatism between nurse educators who belong predominantly to the American Nurses' Association and to the National League for Nursing, and nurse practitioners who belong to the specialty practice groups.

One outcome that should emerge from the new Federation of nursing organizations is a clearer dialogue between educators and practitioners concerning the needs for continued clinical teaching and how this may be provided. No profession can be true to itself unless there is a deep-felt commitment to increasing knowledge, expanding services, and maintaining excellence. For the individual practitioner this involves lifelong learning with or without legislative mandates. For the educational system of the profession, there is an obligation to provide relevant, timely, and authoritative clinical updating. Nursing must face squarely the problems now extant in continuing education for clinical excellence.

## Educational Isolation

The sixth, and final, problem is the parochial separation of our educational patterns throughout the health professions. It is not possible to educate student nurses and student physicians apart from each other, then expect them to function as members of a health team. Health historians point out that up to 1905 there was less difference than one might think between educational patterns experienced by the "trained nurse" and those of the medical student who attended the then current didactic schools of medicine. With the implementation of the Flexner report after 1910, however, medicine moved rapidly into the educational mainstream and nursing remained in the hospital schools. Medical research rapidly expanded the parameters of that profession and the resultant psychologic distance was codified into educational patterns that still remain.

It is time for reexamination of

joint nurse-physician learning at both preparatory, advanced, and continuing levels. The repositioning of nursing education into the collegiate mainstream, the new emphasis on clinical excellence and teacher-practitioner roles, and the establishment of lengthened career perspectives in professional nursing all support a new relationship between the two primary practitioner groups—medicine and nursing.

It was no accident that the AMA and ANA worked together to establish the National Joint Practice Commission between medicine and nursing, or when that body designated a committee to explore educational patterns to foster the joint provision of care by nurses and physicians. There is a "blowin' in the wind" that presages a new relationship between medicine and nursing, one that should be encouraged by nurse educators and practitioners.

## Conclusion

These are educational problems that can and must be solved. Nursing is not granted any luxury in time to set about the work of repatterning and reconstruction. There has been a great deal of talk over the past 50 years; now is the time for concerted and decisive action.

Not all the problems of specialty nursing care, of course, can be attributed to educational difficulties. It wasn't an educator that created utilization patterns for hospital nursing which move nurses inevitably farther and farther away from patient care and more and more closely into administrative systems and paper management. It wasn't an educator who fostered the practice patterns that permit (as in the Yale—New Haven Study) 60 percent of patient care to be provided by untrained aides, attendants, and volunteers while nurses stand atop a pyramidal structure and provide "care through others." These are matters which nurse practitioners must correct. To start, the responsibility for excellence in practice must be reclaimed by the nursing profession.

Education and practice must join hands to ensure that nursing becomes a full profession. A rational pattern of education, fully articulated, clinically excellent, with opportunity for specialty choice, and continuing, interdisciplinary learning must be ensured. All false and illogical barriers by which nurse educators have become isolated and weakened must be eliminated. Client care must become the standard of measurement for the profession and education and research established as the means to that end, not treated as independent entities. It must be demonstrated to the American public and to congruent health practitioners that nursing is capable of facing up to the facts and of taking vital corrective action, no matter what the weight of tradition or the inertia of the status quo.

The author's position on accountability is a distillation of over twenty years' experience as a nurse practitioner, educator and researcher. As a member of the Task Force that developed the Michigan Nurses' Association Position on Nursing Practice, she helped incorporate accountability as one of four critical attributes of the nurse practitioner.

# ACCOUNTABILITY: MYTH OR MANDATE?

*Joyce Y. Passos*

**Joyce Y. Passos, R.N., Ph.D.,** is a lecturer in nursing, Boston State College, Boston, Mass.

Condensed and reprinted with permission from the *Journal of Nursing Administration*, Volume III, Number 3, (May–June 1973), pp. 17–22. Copyright © 1973 by the Journal of Nursing Administration, Inc.

*". . . we are all accountable to someone,
but except in the case of
the private practitioner of nursing,
that someone is not usually
a recipient of health care."*

This article was adapted from an address delivered May 19, 1972, at Adelphi University for the Elizabeth Palmieri Memorial Lecture Series.

Accountability in nursing practice might be described as the "dues paying" aspect of the increasing emphasis in nursing on greater autonomy and independence for the nurse practitioner. Are those who advocate nursing's accountability engaging in moralistic preaching or is accountability a necessary and achievable characteristic of nursing practice? There are three questions we must consider to make that determination.

1. What is the nature of accountability?
2. Why might a nurse aspire to possess this attribute?
3. What else do we need to know about accountability to move this attribute from dream to reality as a necessary characteristic of the nurse practitioner?

## WHAT IS THE NATURE OF ACCOUNTABILITY?

The Position on Nursing Practice approved by the Michigan Nurses' Association defines accountability as "the responsibility for the services one provides or makes available." In a legalistic sense, however, accountability has a liability dimension that responsibility lacks. If one is accountable, one is *liable to be called to account;* that is, held liable for the extent to which the *actions taken* were consistent with the *responsibilities for which one contracted.* Responsibility expresses the "ought's" or expectations of performance, while accountability implies that our "did's" or actual performance will be judged against some standard of performance.

Peplau gives a succinct definition of accountability: "To be accountable means to answer to someone for something that one *has done* [1]." She describes responsibility as a *"charge to do something* for which one is answerable or accountable to someone [2]." Responsibility, whether assigned or taken, must carry with it *authority,* or the rightful power to act. Power, a term with which we are becoming more and more comfortable, may come from either external or internal sources. Peplau identifies knowledge, the law, the authority of the situation, positional authority, and the authority of the group as sources of power or authority [3]. The authority of the group as a power source takes on special meaning in nursing. Are we ready to function as a group to monitor, evaluate, and improve each other's practice? Evaluation of one's performance by peers is a hallmark of professionalism; it is through this mechanism that the profession is held accountable to society.

Accountability is an accounting made of the productivity of an individual, group, or institution. Evaluation and accountability are not the same thing even though the concepts overlap substantially. Evaluation tends to be an internal process (i.e., conducted by and for the benefit of professional peers), while accountability brings with it "the notion of external judgment."

There has been much discussion recently of Nathan Hershey's recommendation that licensure of individuals be restricted to dentists and physicians and that all other health practitioners be licensed by institutions. Unless we are willing to be accountable to those whom we serve, institutional licensure is the only route we can go. Right now it *is* institutions that are held accountable, since the issue of accountability as a necessary attribute for professional nursing practice hinges on whether we are answerable, under the law, for actions we take with pa-

tients. Virginia Driscoll, Executive Director of the New York State Nurses' Association, has spoken of the need to strengthen the present system of individual licensure as a defense against the erosion of nursing as a necessary and identifiable service.

## WHY MIGHT NURSES ASPIRE TO POSSESS ACCOUNTABILITY

There are three motivations which might lead nurses to demonstrate accountability. The first is *idealism,* a belief that "that's the way it should be," a part of the nurse's value system about being in a helping profession. An idealistic conviction about accountability may be separate from any consideration of financial or other rewards. The second motivation is *pragmatism.* Nurses may believe that without being accountable to the individual to be helped, you cannot define his goals and help him to achieve them. The third motivation is *expediency.* Nurses will be accountable if the financial and other rewards are contingent upon the resulting state and satisfaction of those they serve. While I believe that other strategies are more desirable, expediency can produce the desired results, if that is the route we have to follow.

## WHAT ELSE DO WE NEED TO KNOW ABOUT ACCOUNTABILITY?

To answer this question, nursing must answer these difficult but related questions.

1. To whom are we accountable?
2. For what are we accountable?
3. How will our accountability be manifested?
4. How will our performance be monitored?
5. How will acceptable levels of accountability be determined and then regulated and controlled?

### To Whom Are We Accountable?

Right now, we are all accountable to someone, but except in the case of the private practitioner of nursing, that someone is *not* usually a recipient of health care. We are now highly accountable to both the employer, who is the agency in most instances, and to the physician, who may be the employer or a powerful authority source within the agency. However, if we profess professionalism the only way that standards of acceptable performance can be formulated and applied is by professional peers. First, we must be *willing* to judge the performance of our peers, an uncomfortable task for most women; then we must become expert judges. And, we must soon develop strategies for assigning or using professional nurses which will require that the nurse be responsible to the recipient for the quality of service provided.

### For What Are We Accountable?

Alvan Feinstein's description of professionalism in medicine can be applied to the practice of nursing [4].

The professional practitioner is the one who accepts responsibility for the life and welfare entrusted to him by the patient or family, and who discharges that responsibility by planning the strategy, executing the tactics of the therapeutic care indicated by the presenting needs or problems, evaluating the care and determining with the patient and family when service is no longer needed or desired.

How much of this responsibility does a nurse engaged in direct care assume consistently? I propose that the thing *least* characteristic of nursing practice is the determination with the recipient that service is no longer needed or desired. This is greatly deterred, at least in institutional nursing, by the continuous rotation of nursing personnel among patient care areas and among patients in the same area. Such a pattern of personnel assignment makes a myth of accountability.

The ANA *Code for Nurses* describes ten areas in which we are accountable:

1. Providing services which respect the dignity of man.
2. Safeguarding the individual's right to privacy.

3. Maintaining individual competence in nursing practice, recognizing and accepting responsibility for individual actions and judgments.
4. Safeguarding the patient when his care and safety are affected by incompetent, unethical, or illegal conduct of any person.
5. Using individual competence as a criterion in accepting delegated responsibilities and assigning nursing activities to others.
6. Participating in research activities when assured that the rights of individual subjects are protected.
7. Participating in the efforts of the profession to define and upgrade standards of nursing practice and education.
8. Acting through the professional organization to participate in establishing and maintaining conditions of employment conducive to high-quality nursing care.
9. Working with members of health professions and other citizens in promoting efforts to meet health needs of the public.
10. Refusing to give or imply endorsement to advertising, promotion, or sales for commercial products, services, or enterprises.

## How Will Accountability Be Manifested?

That the profession accepts its accountability will be manifested when it articulates standards of nursing practice. One way to define standards is to describe nurse-patient situations that demonstrate the limits within which nursing practice must fall to be acceptable to the profession and the recipient of care. In order to obtain the data needed to apply standards to practice, we must improve the documentation of nursing care.

## How Will Performance Be Monitored?

There are two types of information that must be retrievable if we are to monitor nursing performance: (1) serial measures of the state and satisfaction of recipients, taken at initiation and termination of contact, and at intervals throughout the period of service; and (2) description of the measures taken by nurses to deal with the needs or problems of recipients served. Efforts to introduce systems for documenting nursing care will go far toward providing both types of information.

## How Will Acceptable Levels Be Determined and then Regulated and Controlled?

If we wish to control our own practice, we must conduct peer evaluation. There are many problems associated with this mechanism of control. Some of these are:

1. Facing the issue of trust
2. Relating professional standards, developed by peers, to the policies and procedures which govern settings where nurses practice.
3. Closing the gap between actual practice and the boundaries of practice defined in nursing practice acts

4. Respecting the confidentiality of recipient data, which must be dealt with in peer review in any type of "audit" procedure.
5. Helping nurses to accept the *lack* of anonymity of their performances — an individual must be identifiable if one is to monitor and evaluate her level of practice.
6. Cost analyzing nursing contribution at differential levels of quality.

If we fail to concern ourselves with the means by which manifest nurse behavior can be monitored and regulated, then there is no point in talking about accountability in nursing practice. Our dilemma in trying to isolate this attribute within the nursing process is due in part to the fact that nursing is a social process in which human beings are continually interacting with other human beings in ways that are imperfectly measurable.

The contribution of accountability to nursing practice can be illustrated by an analogy to travel. There are three necessary elements for any successful motor trip: fuel to supply the power; an engine to provide the thrust; and a destination which determines how much fuel and what kind of engine. When the trip is our pilgrimage toward professionalism, the nature of the problems for which we are responsible to society is analogous to the destination; the nature of our services, or treatment modalities, is analogous to the engine, and accountability is analogous to the fuel — it supplies the power.

## REFERENCES

[1] Peplau, H. Responsibility, Authority, Evaluation and Accountability of Nursing in Patient Care. *Michigan Nurse* 44:5–8; (1971).
[2] *Ibid.*
[3] *Ibid.*, p. 8
[4] Feinstein, A. R. *Clinical Judgment.* Baltimore: Williams and Wilkins Co.. 1967, p. 21.

*"We are all familiar with
those individuals and groups
who either do not recognize
the nature of the nursing process
or appreciate it keenly and,
therefore, seek to control it."*

# BEWARE the CIRCLING OPPORTUNISTS

*Veronica M. Driscoll*

In keeping with its historical propensity for flexibility the nursing profession is currently experiencing another phase of functional change. Once again the exquisite adaptability of the nursing process is being tested in an effort to meet health care demands. Nursing practitioners are increasingly employing or being prepared to employ "new" tools, techniques and therapeutic approaches in their provision of nursing care services. In the past, nurses took the initiative in using such tools of the time as the thermometer, sphygmomanometer, intramuscular injection, intravenous therapy and technolo-

**Veronica M. Driscoll, R.N., M.A.** is executive director of The New York State Nurses' Association and editor of its journal.

Reprinted through courtesy of the *Journal of the New York State Nurses' Association,* Volume 4, Number 1, (July 1973), pp. 5–6.

gical devices of diverse complexity. Today's practitioners, no less sensitive to their responsibilities, are including in their repertoire of skills, history taking, physical assessment and prescription of a variety of therapeutic measures. In short, as health science and technology evolve, so does nursing — and practitioners continue to refine their efforts to diagnose and treat human responses to actual or potential health problems.

No one in nursing faults such functional evolution, for it merely confirms the fact that full and appropriate exercise of the nursing process is fundamental to an effective health care delivery system. Therefore, the nursing profession can and will tolerate shifting directions in order to guarantee public access to its vital services. However, what we do object to strenuously is the marked confusion and conflict surrounding the profession's latest change phase. Typically, as nursing takes one step forward a host of circling opportunists seeks to thrust it two steps backward. We are all familiar with these opportunists — those individuals and groups who either do not recognize the nature of the nursing process or appreciate it keenly and, therefore, seek to control it.

As the practice of nursing evolves, confusion and conflict are demonstrated and created by the opportunists with each acquisition by nursing practitioners of some new tool or technique. Consider, for example:

1. Attempts to redefine essential components of the nursing process as exclusively "medically-delegated functions" or "data collection services";
2. Attempts to restrain, intimidate or control nursing practitioners through frequent and hysterical recourse to new "legal opinions" from diverse sources;
3. Attempts to create "new" titles for nursing practitioners to denote their involvement in something other than nursing;
4. Attempts to lure nursing practitioners into medically-dominated roles by labelling new tools and techniques as medically-delegated and supervised and offering attractive economic rewards to nurses willing to function in these capacities, and;
5. Finally, the persistent, insidious attempts to certify nursing prac-

titioners in their evolving role as physician's assistants and to register nursing education programs as physician assistant programs.

In our judgment, the nursing community can resolve all this unfortunate confusion and conflict through reliance on a mere handful of professional guidelines:

1. The responsibility and authority to define or redefine the practice of nursing rests solely with the nursing community.
2. New legal opinions are both unnecessary and inappropriate in view of the fact that there exists in New York State a legal definition of nursing practice which clearly authorizes employment of such tools and techniques.
3. "What's in a name?. . ." "Sticks and stones . . ." "a rose by any other name . . ." . . . the moral is, A nursing practitioner practices *nursing.*
4. Genuine collaboration between and among independent health care practitioners assumes equality of all, not dominance by one.
5. If nursing is to survive as an independent and distinct health profession it cannot be an "either this or that" entity.

In conclusion, we would say to the nursing community, "Beware the circling opportunists" — and carry on!

# Overuse
# of Antibiotics

*Calvin M. Kunin,*
*Thelma Tupasi,*
*and William A. Craig*

At a hearing on the misuse of antibiotics in Washington, D.C., in 1972, Senator Gaylord Nelson stated that "antibiotics are among the most frequently prescribed drugs in this country. The Drug Research Board of the National Academy of Science–National Research Council has also expressed concern about the overprescribing of drugs by physicians. We will review here the evidence that there is such a problem, and offer some solutions. While this subject has been reviewed many times, there has been little overall change in prescribing practices.

"Market research data shows
that about 95 percent of physicians
issue prescriptions to a
patient suffering from the common cold;
almost 60 percent of these
prescriptions are for antibiotics."

**Calvin M. Kunin, M.D.** is chief, Medical Service, Veterans Administration Hospital, Madison, Wisconsin.

**Thelma Tupasi, M.D.** is currently with the Makati Medical Center, Department of Infectious Disease, Makati, Rival, Philippines.

**William A. Craig, M.D.** is assistant chief, Infectious Diseases, Veterans Administration Hospital, Madison, Wisconsin.

Condensed and reprinted with permission from *Annals of Internal Medicine*, Volume 79, Number 4, (October, 1973), pp. 555–560. Nursing Digest assumes full responsibility for the condensation of this article.

## THE PROBLEM

The patterns of antibiotic use and the problems they produce are quite different in hospital and in office practice. In office practice the agents used most frequently are the broad- to medium-spectrum oral agents (tetracyclines, penicillins, erythromycin, and lincomycin), mostly for respiratory infections.

The sporadic use of antibiotics in office practice probably has not had a major effect on the ecology of invading microorganisms, except in individual patients who have been given intense treatment. The reverse is true in hospitals, where Gram-negative enteric bacteria have largely replaced the staphylococcus as the leading cause of bacteremia, just as the staphylococcus replaced the pneumococcus and group A streptococcus in the past two decades.

We are concerned with these developments for the following reasons:

1. The rising costs of medical care are aggravated by overuse of expensive agents. These costs can only be justified by real need.

2. The change in the ecology of hospital infections caused by intensive antibiotic use has had a devastating effect. Investigators recently calculated that Gram-negative bacteremia occurs in approximately 1% of hospitalized patients annually, with a fatality rate of 30% to 50%, or 100,000 fatalities each year.

3. Untoward toxic effects of antibiotics are well known; they range from death from anaphylaxis or aplastic anemia, with penicillin and chloramphenicol, respectively, to severe diarrhea from lincomycin, rash from ampicillin, and nephrotoxicity and ototoxicity from the aminoglycosides.

### Evidence of Overuse

*Office Practice:* Market research data shows that about 95% of physicians issue prescriptions to a patient suffering from the "common cold;"

almost 60% of these prescriptions are for antibiotics. They also found that recently trained doctors who had more postgraduate training used drugs more appropriately.

Dr. Harry Dowling, formerly chairman of the Department of Medicine at the University of Illinois, reported that the FDA certified for fiscal year 1972 about 2,400,000 kg of the eight most commonly used antibiotics, enough to treat two illnesses of average duration for every man, woman, and child in this country. He estimated, however, that the average person has an illness requiring antibiotic treatment no oftener than once every 5 or 10 years. Furthermore, the production of antibiotics for medicinal purposes, in the decade from 1960 to 1970, has increased 320%, and the total cost of antibiotics to hospitals in this country rose 130% during the same time period.

*The Hospital:* Two studies that evaluated the use of antibiotics in community hospitals reached conclusions which were similar: In the first study 62% of the patients who received antibiotics showed no evidence of infection at all; in the second, 65.6% of the patients either required no therapy or received an inappropriate dose.

In another study conducted in 1969 at a university hospital, medication charts of the medical and surgical services were reviewed for all newly admitted patients during a

3-month period. The use of antibiotics was judged in each case according to the best knowledge of the infectious disease resident and two members of the infectious disease group, and by reviewing specific recent literature. The reviewers believed that in 51.5% of patients therapy was either not indicated or the choice of drug or dose was inappropriate. Misuse was more common on surgical than medical services.

## Emergence of the "Drugs of Fear"

Remarkably effective drugs that are active against penicillinase-resistant staphylococci and enteric Gram-negative bacteria, including *Pseudomonas*, have been introduced during the past 5 to 10 years and are now widely used. Unfortunately, although many lives have been saved by these drugs, the conditions that predispose to infection with "difficult hospital bacteria" have not been resolved, and often the drugs have been used either unnecessarily or have simply delayed fatality from infection. Antibiotics seldom prevent or cure infection in the immunosuppressed or anatomically compromised host, and their prophylactic value is overrated.

The availability of the new agents combined with aggressive "education" programs by the pharmaceutical industry has changed the approach of physicians to the care of ill patients and patients in whom infection is only threatened. The physican tends to resort to overuse of these powerful and expensive agents. If he performed a few simple tests and recognized the limitations of antibiotics, the possibility of failure would be greatly lessened, and the patient would be spared toxic hazards and unnecessary expense.

A survey of the use of antimicrobial agents in a university hospital, a Veterans Administration Hospital, and a community hospital was conducted in 1972 to examine the magnitude of the problem and to update a study that was published when the major new drugs were first introduced.

At the Veterans Administration Hospital, we noticed a widespread use of cephalexin, and decided to undertake a control program there. A consultation from the infectious disease service was required before the drug was released from the pharmacy. Although there was a marked increase in use of cephalexin shortly after its introduction, a prompt and almost complete cessation of use occurred after institution of control. No major rise in the use of other agents accompanied the decreased use of cephalexin. The drug simply had not been needed in most cases.

Trends of parenteral antibiotic use at the university hospital during a 2-year period were next examined. These data showed that three drugs were the main contributors to use and cost—cephalothin, gentamicin, and methicillin. Increases in use and expenditure were occurring when the hospital census was falling and despite the fact that pharmacists were stationed on *wards* as therapeutic consultants and dispensers of drugs.

These data on changes in antibiotic use, together with the studies of the quality of decisions on prescribing antibiotics, indicate that the use of antibiotics in hospitals is a major problem.

## WAYS TO IMPROVE USE OF ANTIBIOTICS

The use of antibiotics would be improved by advice from specialists in an infectious disease group and support from an effective diagnostic bacteriology facility. This ideal situation may exist in a few institutions, but even in these the work load is enormous. However, an opinion from infectious disease specialists or consultation with an informed colleague before using an expensive antibiotic would result in major savings for the patient.

At the University of Wisconsin Medical Center we have put the following plan into effect.

1. Hospital infection control has been strengthened, principally by the extensive use and support of a nurse epidemiologist and a strong infection control committee. It is far more important to prevent hospital-acquired infections than to try to treat them.

2. The functions of the diagnostic bacteriology laboratory are made more relevant to the day-to-day care of patients.

3. The teaching of infectious disease is combined with medical microbiology, to correlate basic science with good practice.

4. We are attempting to control the use of expensive antimicrobials.

5. We would like to minimize prophylactic antibiotic routines in the surgical service.

6. A strong drug formulary system is maintained, and the staff is alerted to the complications of antibiotic therapy.

7. We continuously educate students, house staff, and practicing physicians in the use of drugs.

8. We work with community pharmacists to improve prescribing practices by developing a community formulary and continuous monitoring of drug usage.

Let us also recognize that the problem is more broad than simply the use of antibiotics. We are now in an era of explosion in the use of all drugs. In our opinion, medical education programs must be totally independent of the pharmaceutical industry. The education program of the physician must emphasize clinical and laboratory skills and the rational use of drugs. The physician must always be prepared to defend his use of drugs before his peers and must maintain a detached view of their efficacy.

*Abridged from* The Sciences, Volume 13, Number 4, June, 1973.
Joan Solomon © 1973 The New York Academy of Sciences.

# Health Care:
# A Buyer's Market?

Joan Solomon

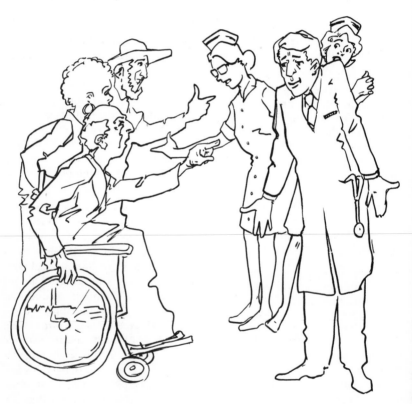

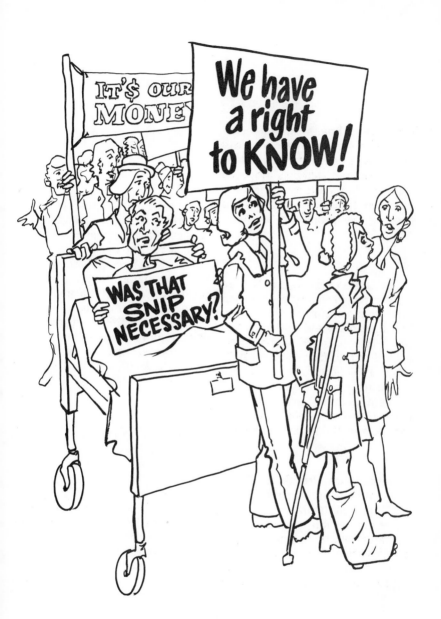

91

The price of health care has risen sharply over the past decade. Health care cannot be boycotted, but consumer activists hope to bring medical costs into line: they want the treatment of disease to become the promotion of well-being.

The United States spends more money per capita on health than any other country in the world. The nation's health bill exceeded $83.4 billion in 1972 and is expected to hit $100 billion by 1975; since 1960, the cost of a day in the hospital has gone up 204 per cent, doctors' fees 74 per cent. People are demanding that health care be a right, not a privilege.

Henry Jones, President of Massachusetts Blue Cross, says, ". . . the health industry . . . has made incredible advances in human skills and technology . . . [But] its actual *delivery system* . . . has made little or no progress during the past few decades and, in some cases, has even retrogressed."

The United States shows up poorly in such telling health indices as infant mortality and life expectancy. The health system fails to meet the needs of the patient," says a major health insurance plan official, who is also a former hospital administrator. "It is left too much to the medical profession to police themselves, to educate themselves. . . . So there are many examples of bad care, of unnecessary care."

Militant consumers point out that the health system is a profit-making industry. Writes a founder of the consumer-professional Medical Liberation Front, "It's simpler and more profitable for the doctor to prescribe the wrong treatment, forcing the patient to return, than to take the time to make the right diagnosis. There's no profit in curing, only in treating—and treating—and treating."

A number of studies indicate that tonsils, uteruses and other organs are often removed needlessly. Pennsylvania Insurance Commissioner Herbert Denenberg recently estimated that only 12 million of the approximately 14 million operations performed each year may really be indicated. In 1960, the Columbia University School of Public Health, studying surgery on 238 families found that 20 of 60 hysterectomies were unnecessary and six more were questionable; seven of 13 Caesarian sections were seriously questioned.

One study showed that prepaid group health care in England and Wales, which offers no economic incentive to perform unnecessary operations, reduces their occurrence drastically.

To combat surgeons whom Commissioner Denenberg calls "knife-happy, incompetent and greedy," some unions have instituted compulsory consultation; the Distributive Workers Union, for example, does not reimburse members fully if they refuse to get a second opinion before surgery. Commissioner Denenberg's diagnosis: "The medical care system . . . is designed by and for hospitals, by and for doctors. . . . Their code of ethics is to keep the truth from the public, and not to tell on one another."

His treatment: holding up rate increases to force medical third parties to set more stringent standards for insurance-covered health care; and publishing and distributing shoppers' guides to health care. This action has won him the enmity of some doctors, lawyers and insurers but, in a recent poll, Pennsylvanians overwhelmingly named him as the state official doing the best job.

## Fraternal Malpractice

Melvin Belli, one of the first lawyers to try malpractice cases, has strong opinions about medical men. "Not every physician gives A-1 care," but the real problem is the cover-up by the good ones of the bad ones." He does not believe in consumer control of medical delivery but suggests that medical professionals should be restricted through publicity, legislation and court actions.

However, according to a recent report of the President's Commission on Medical Malpractice, only 41 per cent of patient-claimants received any payment—although insurers themselves judged that 46 per cent of the claims were "legally meritorious in terms of liability." Half the paid claimants collected less than $3,000, 96 per cent less than $50,000—although 18 per cent of the claims involved death and 19 per cent permanent disability. The Commission's report strongly emphasized the necessity of improving the health care delivery system.

In the 1960s, consumers began to realize that group action was required to improve health delivery. Many consumer health groups are also women's groups. Women make, on the average, 25 per cent more visits to the mostly male doctor population than men do. "The health system is absolutely sexist," contends Pam Booth, a worker at the Women's Medical Center, a New York City health information and counseling organization. "Men run those institutions, whether office or hospital or clinic." "Women are treated as little children," she emphasized.

The main impetus behind the women's medical movement was the fight for abortion reform. Says Rachel Fruchter, who is active in New York City's Women's Health Organizing Collective and a student at the Columbia University School of Public Health, ". . . the abortion experience . . . was devastating not only because of the pain and the illegality, but because it made women realize if they had more money, they would get better care. In this way, it was a distorted but real reflection of the entire health system."

"Most of the women we saw couldn't afford to fly to Puerto Rico or pay $1,000 for a therapeutic abortion. When they had illegal abortions, they were often abused verbally or physically. The polite front typical of medical care faded away. This experience galvanized women because it put them outside the system."

Women also learned that their physicians were giving them conflicting information, particularly about birth control. "We began to realize that . . . we should be able to make choices on the basis of much more information," Ms. Fruchter said.

## Plans of Attack

The current aim of the Women's Health Organizing Collective is to make the health system less fragmented and more responsive to women's needs. Their most impressive project, *A Guide to Women's Health Services in Lower Manhattan, or How to Get Through the Maze with Our Feet in the Stirrups*, outlines the institutions, the services they offer, where they are and how much they cost. Ultimately, the Collective hopes to influence the institutions themselves.

The Women's Medical Center is trying to unify women into a powerful national health coalition. Their first step will be a newsletter that" . . . talks about what we're doing and what we're thinking and the directions we want to go in, as well as finding out what other women are doing, so we don't duplicate each other's mistakes," Ms. Booth told me.

Although the Women's Health Organizing Collective's first objective is comprehensive obstetrics/gynecology clinics with team health delivery and continuity of care, it also envisions total family care health centers. As their guide to women's health services states: "There are some larger changes we must also fight for—the basic right of patients and health workers to control health services and the right of all people to high quality care."

Health-PAC, founded in New York in 1968 and now also operating in California, publishes monthly bulletins analyzing various aspects of the heatlh care system.

"The system must be accountable to consumers," says Ms. Susan Reverby, a staff member of Health-PAC. "It's their money and their bodies, and that should give them ultimate control over health institutions." Worker control is also crucial, she maintains. "You need the people on the inside to feed you information, to help you understand, to be part of the policy-making machinery."

One of the main developments with which consumers must deal is the corporatization of medicine. Power currently lies with medical superstructures. The AMA is shrinking in resources and prestige; hospitals and medical centers, connected through vast networks of affiliations, have become medical empires. Power also resides in the financial-planning complex, particularly Blue Cross, and in the alliance between health care providers and such industrial organizations as drug companies, hospital supply companies, hospital construction companies and banks. "Last, but far from least," says Dr. Kunnes of the Medical Liberation Front, "are major governmental planning boards, agencies, and departments, including the Department of Defense."

One health administrator admits the existence of a complex and powerful medical system, but he says "it is not a structured, organized phenomenon with inter-locking directorates, collusions, antitrust suits. Everyone is simply doing their own thing."

Undoubtedly though, government is trying to gain some control over the private medical system, and consumer participation is being mandated by both Federal and state legislation.

## Consumer Boards

However, some community boards include as consumers members of the hospital Board of Trustees, and individuals appointed by the hospital, not elected by the community. A member of Brooklyn's Methodist Hospital's Ambulatory Care Services Advisory Committee, mandated by New York State's Ghetto Medicine Act, told of the difficulties in influencing hospital policy. "You don't understand half of what they're saying, and every time you bring up something you want to improve, they say there's not enough money. Some hospitals have controlled boards, but we try to make things tough. For everything we want, we hassle, we cajole, we demand, we write letters to the press." Their most potent power: if the board advises the Department of Health of non-compliance with Ghetto Medicine guidelines, the hospital loses money.

Efforts to create a national consumer health movement have failed because of factionalization and splitting. Local groups may work at cross-purposes because they are not in touch with each other.

Also hampering the consumer movement are inevitable arguments. As a city official in health planning put it, "When consumer groups are splintered, they become ineffective. Providers won't respond to their demands."

## Struggles of a Free Clinic

In opposition to consumers who would challenge existing institutions are those who would set up alternate ones—most often, free clinics. Since the Haight-Ashbury Free Clinic opened in San Francisco in 1967, hundreds more have been formed throughout the country. They aim to give good health care in untraditional ways for little or no money. Most of them experiment with community/worker control and stress the transfer of skills as a way to demystify and deprofessionalize medicine.

Detractors in the consumer movement say, "They don't provide decent care . . . because they're on a tenuous funding basis. Ultimately they fragment care because they can only provide bits and pieces."

Advocates of free clinics reply that they are models and instruments for change—and they *do* provide good care. At a free clinic on New York's lower east side, patients are usually young adults who have gynecologic, dermatologic or minor medical problems. "They don't want the rigamarole, the red tape, the hassle of a hospital clinic," said a registered nurse who does volunteer work at the clinic.

"The best medicine I've ever seen practiced happens here. I was trained in a city hospital. The patients would wait for two hours and then be rushed through in five minutes. Here, if they need a half hour, we give them a half hour. The physicians and other workers are kind and sensitive." Although the Free Clinic is struggling for financial survival, it hopes to add counseling and social services.

Another medical consumer split is between "radicals," who want a total restructuring of the medical delivery system and a total shift of power, and "reformists," who would be satisfied with consumer input. New York's Comprehensive Health Planning

97

Agency—a coalition of consumers and providers—is a reformist group. Created out of the Federal Partnership for Health Act, a 1966 amendment to the Public Health Law, it is part of New York City government; consumer members, who constitute a one-person majority, were selected from already existing citywide groups.

One member, a union official, thinks it's "healthy" to have a consumer majority. But he would *not* like to see consumer control. "Consumers should be consulted and involved, but they can't direct physicians or hospital Boards of Directors. There must be a partnership."

Most health care providers give lip service to consumerism, but point out what they consider its dangers. "All too often, consumers are well-intentioned, but just don't know what it is to take care of patients or to get care delivered," states a health insurance official.

Dr. Cherkasky of Montefiore would like to see a team effort between professional people who know the instrument and lay people who are socially concerned. "The more thoughtful the community leadership, the sooner we'll achieve that day."

## The Most Vital Consumer Weapon

One very thoughtful medical consumerist is Edward Gluckmann, executive vice-president of the Consumer Commission on the Accreditation of Health Services, a consumer information service. Mr. Gluckmann sees his organization as a countervailing force to the Joint Commission on the Accreditation of Hospitals; the board of *that* Commission is composed only of providers and its accreditation programs are financially supported by the surveyed hospitals.

In three to five years, he says, consumer commissions in every major city may be publicizing heretofore secret information, demanding the right to monitor health care delivery, and "making the damn system a little more responsive and accountable to the people who pay the bills." Mr. Gluckmann also wants to form an organization to educate consumers in the politics of health.

Education is now critical to the medical consumer movement. Consumers who want to make their partnership with providers meaningful must begin to counteract charges of ignorance.

# Old Professionals
# In A New World

*by Per G. Stensland*

Ours has become a society dominated by professionals. The famous ancient trilogy of learned professions — theology, law and medicine — has long been replaced by a formidable list of special occupations. Common usage, like Webster, has bestowed the name on all those groups of people who claim to have acquired "some special knowledge used by way of either instructing, guiding, or advising others or serving them in some art." The setting and the task of all these professionals have altered dramatically, since they acquired the "special knowledge." This is a commentary on the old professional in a new world.

The horizontal dimension of profession has changed: the society in which most professions were born is gone, the present setting is in violent change.

**Per G. Stensland, Ph.D.**, is senior associate for the Milbank Memorial Fund, New York, New York 10005.

Condensed and reprinted with permission from *Adult Leadership,* (April, 1973), Volume 21, Number 10, pp. 315-317. Copyright © 1973 by the Adult Education Association of the U.S.A.

Simultaneously, the vertical dimension has changed: the knowledge and skill that were so special when most professionals now active went to school have lost their validity.

In this setting, professions face either conflict or accommodation, death or rebirth. We urgently need to take a fresh look at the nature and role of professions. Five years ago, I placed an optimistic choice before a group of registered nurses in Canada: "Whether there shall be an open collision or not, there will no doubt be an increasingly pressing demand for leadership to use all human resources, professional and non-professional in constant work on building a new world and adjusting or changing the old patterns to fit new conditions. In this business of construction and reconstruction, education will play a central role."

I still believe in an open choice and am optimistic, but I fear that professional education requires far bolder ideas and sharper assessment than we have come up with since 1966. We need to produce a new professional, not just an updated old one. That new professional is the doctor, nurse, lawyer, journalist, engineer, teacher, social worker, clergyman, or city planner with new insights, competencies, and commitments fitted for future work together with people only recently regarded as colleagues.

## THE NATURE AND ROLE OF PROFESSIONS

Four characteristics of professions are worth noting:

First, professions are created by a basic need for the peculiar form of work. The basic justification for a profession is service to others. This distinguishes the professional occupations from the scientist whose basic justification is pursuit of knowledge or the business man whose prerogative is commerce or work.

The assertion is in the professions that you and no one else can best give the service you give, and that people need that service. However, the needs are fluid and shifting, particularly in the so-called "helping professions."

Second, professionals are not just another group of working people, rendering service to meet needs. They are unique in the sense that they are expected to operate with technical competence in restricted areas under generally accepted standards. To these criteria may be added objectivity and priority for clients.

Third, professions are largely self-regulating. Some of them, like physicians, have a legally supported monopoly, with a special kind of authority much like the limits bureaucrats set on customers.

Fourth, some professions, notably the medical, have a peculiar autonomy. This has put a few powerful tools in their hands: monopoly over performance through licensure, control of production and application of knowledge and skill, and a code of ethics.

These four characteristics make it obvious that very often it is the professional not the system that controls how well the basic needs are being met and services performed. In the field of health care it is the doctor not the system, the technology or the money that dominates. The physician holds the key to how well, where, and whether health services are delivered.

## THE NEW PROFESSIONAL TASK

Professionals like the rest of us are now facing a revolutionary upheaval in four areas of human life. First, physically, we are in the midst of a new major settlement shift — of equal importance to the great change from nomadic hunting 10,000 years ago. What man started to build then — home communities — is no longer real.

The revolutionary change in the environment has profoundly altered the world of work for the new professionals. They need to be involved in the new community that is the world in which they all work. No more can the new doctor deal with individual patients than he can deal with individual organs.

To be truly effective, the new professional needs to understand the total community environment. He needs to understand the dynamic processes of change and the nature of development. The physician, the engineer, the clergyman, and the lawyer share with unexpected new colleagues a profound stake in the destiny of a new world, where special insights and skills have little meaning unless they fit the larger community.

Second, human relationships have changed with the advance of science in the matter of communication and cooperation. We now are able to talk and listen to anyone anywhere, and we have gained insights into how we may more effectively talk and listen to each other.

As the new professionals are facing a revolution in human relationships, they must build new patterns of cooperation. In the world of health, the doctor so far has been in a privileged position. Facing a world of new relationships, though, the doctor needs to move toward cooperation and shared power. Some time ago, Lawrence Frank called on professional workers of every kind to "accept this urgent need for joint exploration and concerted efforts to develop a more acceptable common understanding in all their specialized work."

Mere changes in education are not enough. Professional roles must be redefined, barriers between professions broken down, new channels of communication opened up.

The third area of revolutionary change is in intellectual resources. Scientific discovery and technological production have immensely enlarged our scope for action. Our technological capacity is so incredible that we now probably are able to provide for all the needs of mankind to live, and all the means to die.

In the face of explosive increase in knowledge, the new professional will have to be able to cope with the new technical and intellectual resources. The computer has opened new unheard of possibilities for him to gather, store, analyze and disseminate information, for diagnosis as well as didactics. Electronics have radically changed his communications through satellites, television, highpowered new microscopes, or surgical instruments. He must learn to let machines perform tasks for which he once acquired now obsolete competencies.

The effective utilization of new resources, ideas and innovations is, of course, not automatic. It requires reshaped professional education — not through mechanical curriculum shifts but through radical change in teaching/learning experiences, through rethinking of the role of the professor, and of the university.

Finally, we are probably in a major shift of values and ideals, equal to the great push 500 years ago. Excitements and commitments in the Western world are being violently challenged by both Westerners and Easterners. Notions about cause and effect, work and leisure, nation and world, love and hate, God and man, myself and others are under deep and constant scrutiny. There are no longer any sacred ideas, things, people or cows.

The new professional must feel at

home with this revolution in values. In the area of general wellbeing of mankind, the new doctor must be hospitable to the dramatic shift in ideas and ideals about basic human phenomena: birth, death, ecology, money, drugs, life goals. He must dare to lead, not dominate, contribute to the search for new knowledge and new use of old, innovate rather than inculcate, explore rather than exploit.

In the world of health, the new professional must boldly participate in creating a new professional ethics that provides consistent responses to questions like these: how can one develop adequate trust in fellow professionals, in clients, in patients, customers, government? How can one build structures and organizations flexible enough to accommodate intellectual and technical innovations? How can one acquire a sense of joint responsibility for finding adequate data and information about the world around us? Finally, how can one break patterns for new controls and moral principles serving a life less authority bound, less obedience ridden, less fearful of fellowmen, more truly optimistic about the future.

Francis Bacon once said "I hold every man a debtor to his profession; from the which as men of course do seek to receive countenance and profit, so ought they of duty to endeavor themselves by way of amends to be of help and ornament thereunto." Hearing this distant voice from the early hours of our modern scientific age, the new professional must realize that his "help and ornament" is not only to old colleagues, but to new ones, indeed to mankind around him.

Condensed and reprinted from *PRISM* magazine, Volume 1, Number 6, (September, 1973), pp. 19–61. Copyright © 1973 by the American Medical Association.

# Let's Get the Nurse's Role into Focus

*Unless physicians and nurses recognize the need for flexibility in their professional relationships, says the author, society will brand both groups obsolete.*

*Eleanor C. Lambertsen*

**Eleanor C. Lambertsen, Ed.D.** is dean and professor, Cornell University-New York Hospital of Nursing.

The controversy over the changing role of nurses in health care services has become so bitter in recent years that it is almost impossible to discuss the subject rationally.

Much of the furor derives from the competing claims of two powers —physicians and nurses. Role blurring has been a continuing phenomenon throughout the evolution of the physician-nurse relationship. Recognition of the interdependence of all who serve society's health needs should be the motivating force in any redefinition of professional responsibilities.

## Bored with Promises

A significantly increasing number of nurses and physicians believe that unless both professions objectively face up to the issues related to scope of practice, both groups will be branded obsolete. In this era of people power, the consumer is bored with promises and demonstrably hostile toward those who fail to produce.

103

In 1970, a multidisciplinary HEW committee studied extended roles for nurses. The committee's report outlined the elements of nursing practice under three major segments of the delivery system: primary care, acute care, and long-term care.

It seems clear, from the extended roles envisioned by the committee, that selected nurses will increasingly function as principal health care practitioners in providing community health services directed toward health maintenance, protection against disease and disability, as well as services for the chronically ill and aged. The role of the nurse in acute phases of illness or disability may be either contributing or supportive, for, in these circumstances, the physician is indeed the principal health care practitioner.

## Nursing Functions

In my view, nursing functions encompass care supportive to life and well being and include the following: case findings, diagnostic assessment, teaching about health, individual or family health counseling, therapeutic intervention (psychological or physiological), and restorative services. But when nurses engage in therapeutic intervention, some purists among them proclaim that they are selling their birthright by accepting tasks delegated by the physician. On the other hand, when they take part in diagnostic assessment, alarmists in medicine proclaim that

nurses are stepping over the boundary into medical practice.

Why is it, I wonder, that if a nurse uses a stethoscope to take a blood pressure reading she is not deemed to be practicing medicine? Or if she uses a stethoscope to listen to the heartbeat of a fetus and thereafter makes some judgments, why is this not questioned? Conversely, when someone suggests that she might use a stethoscope on a person's chest to detect deviations of the heart or lungs, why is it that a chorus of protest arises, claiming this as a medical act? Are certain anatomical areas off limits for nurses?

Perhaps the greatest barrier to understanding the potential scope of nursing practice in health care has been the assumption that all nurses are alike in talent and education. This is, of course, far from the case. Moreover, within the practice of nursing, there is a wide range of functions that vary greatly in complexity.

At the risk of sounding simplistic, registered nurses currently in practice may be classified into two groups: (1) those who are prepared to function within existing patterns of practice; and (2) those who are prepared to function within unstructured or ambiguous patterns.

## Areas of Responsibility

I believe that practicing physicians and nurses are well aware of the determinants that differentiate their areas of responsibility. Let us look at the requirements for health services preceding, during, and following a pregnancy. They illustrate a model of nursing and medical practice that is equally applicable to other areas where nurse and physician function together.

Nurse midwives and public health nurses are assuming major roles in genetic counseling and in family planning clinics. During the prenatal months, the nurse may assume the principal responsibility for health counseling, family counseling, and health maintenance for the individual experiencing a normal pregnancy. But if a deviation from the anticipated course occurs, a physician's services are indicated.

During labor, the nurse monitors the progress of the patient and the status of the fetus in utero, sustains the patient when indicated, and employs appropriate measures of intervention. Here again, the services of a physician are indicated if there is a deviation from the normal or anticipated course of labor.

Likewise, the nurse midwife is capable of the management of a normal or uneventful delivery, but the need for a physician is indicated if there is any potential or predictable interference with the delivery. Following delivery, the nurse may assume primary responsibility for health counseling and health maintenance of the mother and infant and refer to the physician those individuals deviating from the normal course of development.

I have not elaborated on the differences in clinical competence and judgment required for a nurse, a public health nurse, a nurse midwife, a physician, an obstetrician, a gynecologist, or a pediatrician. The complexity of the phenomena encountered at any stage of care clearly indicates the need for either a physician or a nurse with preparation appropriate to meet the situation.

A joint statement aimed at correcting deficits in the availability and quality of maternity care was issued in January, 1971, by the American College of Obstetricians and Gynecologists (ACOG), the Nurses Association of ACOG, and the American College of Nurse Midwifery. It is a significant statement for America, but other countries have long recognized the place of the nurse midwife in their health service system.

Perhaps one of the most important conclusions in the statement is that the deficits in availability and quality of maternity care can best be corrected by the cooperative efforts of physicians, nurse midwives, obstetric registered nurses, and other health personnel. The intent is not to limit the services to any social class, but to recognize that the composition of the health team will vary and be determined by local needs and circumstances. Its functions and responsibilities will be defined according to the education and training of the professionals concerned.

# Training Programs

The Family Nurse Practitioner Program (PRIMEX) is the most recent effort to formalize the expanded role of nurses. Seven projects are preparing registered nurses, through continuing education programs, to function in ambulatory care settings, including outpatient departments, neighborhood health centers, industrial health services, and doctors' office practices, among others. The services are community oriented and related to the needs, concerns, and priorities of consumers.

All of these PRIMEX projects share in the development of protocols to evaluate the effectiveness of the training programs for graduate nurses with a variety of educational backgrounds (associate of arts degree, hospital diploma, baccalaureate and master degrees) and the effectiveness of the practitioners in the health care delivery system.

The programs build upon previous academic and professional experiences and focus on extending the scope of the individual's practice capability. The main emphasis is upon primary care and stabilized chronic illness. With patients who are acutely ill or who evidence an acute episode in a chronic illness, the family nurse practitioner is prepared to make an initial evaluation of the health status and necessary diagnostic procedure. She may then make one of three decisions: (1) intervene immediately with or without medical consultation; (2) arrange for emergency care; or (3) refer the patient to a physician.

Major changes are required in undergraduate and graduate curricula to prepare nurses for expanded roles in the delivery of health services. Moreover, short- and long-term continuing education programs involving schools of nursing and medical schools must be encouraged and endorsed by nurse educators. In more immediate terms, experienced nurses currently in practice, regardless of their educational background, could provide an excellent pool of new practitioners.

A nurse must, of course, be adequately trained to perform competently the particular function required of her; furthermore, she will always be measured—in legal definition by what a reasonably prudent member of her profession would have done under the same, or similar, circumstances. This clearly implies that neither a nurse nor a physician should undertake to make a clinical judgment, institute a course of therapy, or perform a procedure beyond her or his qualifications.

There are no legal barriers to the functions presented in the 1970 HEW report. But since nurse practice acts define practice only in broad terms, a movement has recently developed in a number of states to specify nursing functions more precisely and, in some instances, to redefine them. The critical issue has been the inclusion of the term diagnosis, and its acceptance has involved considerable give-and-take. The New York State Nurses Association, for example, has revised the definition of nursing practice approved by their state legislature in 1972. The revised definition reads, in part, as follows:

## Definition of Nursing Practice

"The practice of the profession of nursing as a registered professional nurse is defined as diagnosing and treating human responses to actual or potential health problems through such services as case findings, health teaching, health counseling, and provision of care supportive to or restorative of life and well being, and executing medical regimens prescribed by a licensed or otherwise legally authorized physician or dentist. A nursing regimen shall be consistent with and shall not vary an existing medical regimen."

Both the New York State Medical Society and the Hospital Association objected to the use of the term "diagnosis," but the conflict was subsequently resolved by defining diagnosis in nursing practice as identification of, and discrimination between, physical and psychosocial signs and symptoms essential to effective execution and management of the nursing regimen. A phrase stating that such diagnostic privilege is distinct from medical diagnosis was also added.

## Social Change

Whatever the precise wording of a specific piece of legislation, it is abundantly clear that current trends in the delivery of safe and effective health care reflect the enormous magnitude of social change in our society. These include changes in science and technology, in social structure, intellectual concepts, and economic and political establishments. The signs and symptoms of social stress are clearly evident in the dissatisfactions of health care consumers, as well as in the changing attitudes of health personnel, regarding the scope, purposes, and rewards of their work. Is it not time that physicians, nurses, and other health-related professionals make determined efforts to attain a high degree of flexibility in their interprofessional relations? I think so.

107

# Psychosurgery, the Courts and Congress

Continuing publicity about psychosurgery
and experimentation on humans
has prompted the courts and Congress
to move toward control

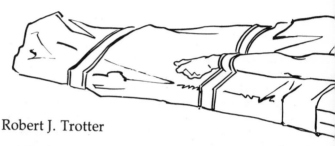

Robert J. Trotter

Mr. L., a 36-year-old mental patient, has lived the last 18 years in Ionia State Hospital in Michigan. He has a history of uncontrollable rages and is alleged to have murdered and then raped a nurse. Mr. L. had little hope of release until he recently volunteered and was selected to take part in a research program. The Lafayette Clinic at Wayne State University in Detroit had received $118,400 from the Michigan legislature to compare psychosurgery to drug therapy as treatments for violent behavior. Mr. L. opted for the surgical procedure, which if successful would allow him to be reintegrated into society. If unsuccessful, he would go back to Ionia.

Before the operation could be performed, however, Gabe Kaimowitz, a Michigan Legal Services lawyer and member of the Medical Committee for Human Rights, found out about it and charged that the patient was being held on an obsolete law, that the circumstances made informed consent impossible and that public funds should not be used for such operations. The case went to court and the patient changed his mind about the operation, claiming he was not fully

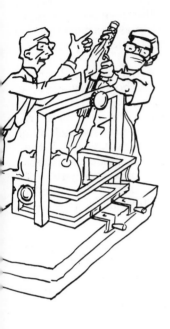

tor in arousing concern and halting (at least temporarily) such attempts at psychosurgery has been the work of Washington psychiatrist Peter R. Breggin. For the past two years he has been preaching long and loud against all forms of psychosurgery. His message has been delivered in person at scientific meetings, in newspapers, magazines and journals, on television in England, in his novels and at great length in the Congressional Record. Breggin's most recent hearing was before the Senate Health Subcommittee, chaired by Sen. Edward M. Kennedy (D-Mass.). Attacking a variety of psychosurgical procedures and practitioners, Breggin charged: "If America ever falls to totalitarianism, the dictator will be a behavioral scientist and the chief of police will be armed with lobotomy and psychosurgery."

informed about the effects of psychosurgery (possible blunting of intellect and emotion). The court ruled that Mr. L. was being held unconstitutionally and ordered his release (although he may now go to prison for murder and rape). The publicity surrounding the case forced the Michigan legislature to withdraw support from the research.

This case illustrates the ethical complexity and increasing public sensitivity toward surgical modification of behavior. A major fac-

Telling the other side of the story were Robert G. Heath of Tulane University and Orlando J. Andy of the University of Mississippi Medical Center. Since 1950 Heath has been developing techniques for implanting electrodes in the brains of patients. His work involves localizing the pathways of emotion and feeling in the brain. Once the pathway is pinpointed, an electrode can be inserted and various feelings (pain or pleasure) can be elicited. He has performed this type of operation on 65 patients, and he emphasized the widespread therapeutic power of such stimulation. He gave an example of two chronic marijuana users. "Since this treatment program was carried out, and since they were stimulated particularly in the pleasure circuitry, neither one of them has wanted to touch marijuana. The pleasure with marijuana did not begin to approach the stimulation of the pleasure sites." Breggin believes the implantation of the electrodes is more destructive than beneficial.

Andy, a major target of Breggin's criticism, told the committee that he has performed 30 to 40 psychosurgery operations since the early 1950's. Of these, 13 or 14 have been on children between the ages of 6 and 19. "We are dealing," he says, "with those patients by far who have been abandoned by the psychiatrists and in many cases have been institutionalized."

Andy said he believes psychosurgery should be used on patients considered to be a detriment to themselves and society. It should be used for custodial purposes when a patient requires constant attention, supervision and an inordinant amount of institutional care. It should be used, he went on, when patients require so much medication that it makes them nonresponsive and noncommunicative. "Finally, it should be used in the adolescent and pediatric age group in order to allow the developing brain to mature with as normal a reaction to its environment as possible."

Many practitioners and proponents of psychosurgery agree, at least in part, with Andy. When the situation meets these requirements and when all other forms of therapy have failed, they feel surgery is indicated. Opponents of psychosurgery ask: "Who is to decide that all other forms of treatment have been tried?"

Neither the medical profession nor the Government imposes any form of control over such operations. The medically ignorant patient must rely on the word of the doctor. Most psychosurgeons do go through elaborate patient selection procedures and most medical facilities maintain close watch over such operations. But all that is really required is consent of the patient, or when that is not possible, consent of the next of kin.

This lack of control was a major topic of discussion at the hearings. Willard Gaylin, president of the Institution of Society, Ethics and the Life Sciences at Hastings-on-Hudson, N.Y., noted that "the kinds of controls in psychosurgery have been casual to the point of irresponsibility." Follow up and peer review have been very poor. Gaylin does not believe psychosurgery should be abandoned but says, "I am not sure it has been given enough safeguards."

In fact, there is no way to prohibit psychosurgery by a private doctor, said Bertram S. Brown, director of the National Institute of Mental Health. Not enough is known, he said, about brain functioning to justify psychosurgical procedures unless there is very strong evidence of organic pathology in the brain.

Brown said the goal of psychosurgery is to pinpoint the locus of undesirable behavior in the brain and destroy only those tissues and nerve cells—leaving other functions and behaviors unaffected. "Frankly," he concluded, "the current practice of psychosurgery falls short of this goal." He called for a study of the estimated 500 annual psychosurgery operations that take place in the United States before any new procedures for overseeing psychosurgery are recommended.

Not everyone, however, is willing to wait for a private study. The Kennedy subcommittee's hearings on psychosurgery, for instance, were only part of six days of hearings on human experimentation and biomedical ethics. More hearings are scheduled, and legislation on the subject is expected to follow shortly from Kennedy. Even if it doesn't, a flurry of legislation has already hit the floors of both the Senate and the House. Much of it deals directly with psychosurgery, but some—spurred by disclosure of the Tuskegee Syphilis Study—deals with the whole area of human experimentation.

It seems apparent that a growing number of legislators feel some sort of controls should be imposed on human experimentation and psychosurgery. Most of the proposed bills apply only to federally funded work, but many lawmakers believe that any forthcoming Federal guidelines would be followed by private practitioners.

This article was taken from Volume 103 of Science News, dated May 12, 1973.

A little twit in a candy-striped uniform, Cherry Ames (who was so named because her cheeks "blazed" every time a handsome young intern passed by), gollyed and gee-whizzed her way through nearly 30 volumes of nursing adventures which undoubtedly influenced the generations that considered Nancy Drew the epitome of glamour and success.

The public, lots of doctors, and even some nurses still view Cherry, Hot Lips (the nympho nurse immortalized in the movie M\*A\*S\*H), and maybe even Florence Nightingale as women who dedicated themselves to selfless duty in order to find a husband, i.e., doctor. As nurses they are expected to treat doctors with wifely obedience, devote a mother's loving care to their patients, and supervise hospital per-

# The Nursing Profession: Condition Critical

**Trucia D. Kushner**

*Trucia D. Kushner* is a free lance writer whose articles have appeared in several national publications, including Ms., New York Magazine and Time-Life. She received a Master's degree in journalism from Boston University.

*Condensed and reprinted with permission from* Ms. Magazine, Volume II, Number 2, (August, 1973), p. 72. Copyright © 1973 by Ms. Magazine.

sonnel with the kindly discipline of a household manager dealing with maids, butlers, and grocery boys. No wonder so many men have the idea that nurses make ideal wives.

Those diehard nursing stereotypes may be breathing their last, however. A new breed of nurses is emerging—a result of the cross-pollination between the Women's Movement and the health-care crisis. Encouraged by the improving status of women, nurses are beginning to see themselves as the obvious answer to huge gaps in this country's health-care system.

Efforts to make nursing separate but equal to doctoring will not only raise the nurse's status, but will ultimately improve patient care. Yet, ironically, the opposition is very strong, magnified in intensity by the femaleness of the nurse role and the maleness of the doctor stereotype.

Take the case of Barbara, 27, who recently began trying to organize nurses where she works. Barbara was "radicalized" when she realized a man she was deeply involved with was putting her down for being a nurse. "It made me so angry that I had to prove myself. Being a nurse was like being a woman; I had to dispel the image that I was just pretty and dumb. As nurses we've all been inculcated with the 'they need me' trip, but I began to realize I had to do something to make my life better. Most people go into nursing because they have the attitude, 'I come last.' That's why we have so much trouble organizing!

Nurses like Barbara pose a tremendous threat to many doctors, as professionals and as men. And on top of these pressures the beleaguered nurse endures competition within the ranks of her own profession since the woman in white is treated the same regardless of the extent of her education or the seriousness of her career goals.

Like her background, the salary and job descriptions of the "nurse" cover a wide spectrum, ranging from $4,000 to $9,000 a year for a practical nurse in a hospital or doctor's office to the $50,000 earned by one select Director of Nursing at a major university.

It seems truly incredible that in the health-care field, which is subdivided into more than 200 job categories, with new ones added all the time, a nurse is a nurse is a nurse. The college-educated nurse often sees herself as a "professional" and regards L.P.N.'s and diploma school R.N.'s as "technicians." But nurses with wide and often painfully acquired experience resent college graduates who start at high salaries before they even learn to make a bed. The L.P.N. category tends to attract more minority women. An American Nursing Association survey in 1968-1969 showed that black women were 3.2 percent of the graduates from R.N. programs, but 15.5 percent of the graduates from L.P.N. programs. Black graduates of baccalaureate R.N. programs actually dropped from 9.7 percent in 1962 to 4 percent in 1966.

The divisions within nursing tend to be functional as well as racial. L.P.N.'s in some states are licensed by boards made up exclusively of R.N.'s. Furthermore, in New York State, where L.P.N.'s do serve on the licensing boards, they are restricted to voting on issues related to L.P.N.'s only, while the R.N.'s can vote on all issues.

One of the most confusing dilemmas faces the nurse who chooses to fulfill the "female comforter" role and remain close to the patient. While this type of one-to-one relationship keeps the hospital operating on a humane scale, it traps the nurse with her own good motives. The more "professional" she becomes (i.e., the further away from the patient), the more money and status she acquires.

**SALARY SCALES**
**(according to ANA)**

| | |
|---|---|
| Nurse's aide | |
| | $3,500 to $7,500 |
| Licensed Practical Nurse | |
| | $4,000 to $9,000 |
| General Staff Nurse (floor duty) | |
| | $5,400 to $12,500 |
| Specialist (for instance, operating room nurse) | |
| | $7,500 to $15,000 |
| Nurse Anesthetist | |
| | $7,500 to $16,400 |
| Head Nurse | |
| | $7,500 to $17,500 |
| Director of Nursing | |
| | $12,500 to $20,000 |
| Dean of School of Nursing | |
| | up to $50,000 |

Historically doctors (read "men") established themselves as *the* legal and official medical profession, when they suppressed and finally outlawed the practice of female "lay" healers, "witches," and spreaders of "old wives' tales." Ever since this active male takeover of the medical profession women have been relegated to a subsidiary position. Nursing was, for years, a job without a legal status of its own.

By the mid-19th century it was a rare woman who was accepted into medical school, or survived the harassments of her "fellow" students. If they made it through to practice, women were excluded from medical associations, and exempted from a male colleague's referral system. Society seemed so set on excluding women from medicine that even midwives, who had functioned since biblical times, were outlawed state by state because they were alleged to be "hopelessly dirty, ignorant, and incompetent." This, despite the findings of a 1912 Johns Hopkins study that most American doctors were less competent than midwives.

Thus discredited even to deliver their own progeny, women were left only one option in health care—to enter nursing. In an era of Victorian morality and abominable hospital conditions, nursing was considered a disreputable occupation.

Conditions constituted a call of duty to reformers like Florence Nightingale (1820-1910), the founder of modern nursing as we know it. But along with that credit, she must also take the blame for endowing the occupation with all the sexist hangups she felt as an aristocratic Victorian lady. She encouraged wellbred young women to emancipate themselves from their subservient role in the home by coming to dispense charity at the hospital. Although it probably seemed a radical move at the time, in retrospect it looks like stepping from one straitjacket into another. Women's hospital duties involved low-paid, heavyduty housework, to be pursued in a "ladylike" fashion, with the emphasis on character rather than skills. The profession has only recently begun to shed such Victorian accessories as standing when a doctor enters the room. Upper- and middle-class values were on the working-class women who were eventually attracted to the profession.

Nightingale greeted the suggestion that nurses, like doctors, be subject to exams and licensing with the comment: "Nurses cannot be registered and examined any more than mothers." By 1923 state licensure was achieved, but even that did not take away the stigma of "woman's work."

The inevitable link between the profession and women's status in society was appreciated by one nurse and early feminist, Lavinia Dock. In 1907, Dock asked the national Nurses Associated Alumnae to pass a resolution endorsing the suffrage movement. Of course, the resolution didn't pass. It was only in 1970 that the American Nurses Association finally endorsed the Equal Rights Amendment, and even then it was approved by the vote of the board of directors, because the convention "never got to it." In order to be fair, it must be said that several state associations —Vermont, Hawaii, Colorado, and others—actively lobbied for passage of the ERA, but in other areas, state associations have been oblivious or unconcerned.

Despite the direct interest nurses have in sex discrimination and women's issues, many nurses resist the feminist movement for fear of being associated with "bra-burners." Some feel slurred by the feminist cliché: "Tell your little girl to be a doctor, not a nurse." Obviously that is not the way to win the support of the nursing profession, although many nurses will privately admit they wish they had gone to medical school.

A former registered nurse, National Organization for Women (NOW) president Wilma Scott Heide comments: "Nursing, in my view and that of feminists and behavioral scientists, reflects the secondary status of women. To the extent that physicians are male and nurses female, you have the prototype of the male-female relationship of the culture at large. The doctor is in charge, the nurse serves."

Nurses were traditionally taught to be submissive, obedient, and feminine in the strictly disciplined environment of the nursing school. The paradox became complete when the responsibility and autonomy they were promised failed to materialize after graduation.

Today, more and more nurses are studying alongside doctors. Nurses are hopeful that this will educate doctors about the intelligence and basic humanity of nurses. But a lot more than classroom exposure may be necessary.

For, while nurses are training in the skills of tact, sensitivity, and diplomacy, medical students are urged in the opposite direction. For doctors, decisiveness and authority are encouraged. The students are told repeatedly that mistakes can mean life or death—so they'd better not make any. In order to function without constant fear and anxiety, the prospective doctor is taught to develop a feeling of omnipotence to prepare for this awesome responsibility. Doctors are totally unprepared to take directions from anyone, least of all "uppity" nurses.

In the hospital setting the male-female role caricature has been called the "doctor-nurse game." The object of the game is to make the doctor feel in control at all times. To do this the nurse must make significant recommendations in such a way that they appear to be initiated by the doctor. She must be actively helpful, yet appear passive. An example of this kind of game was offered by a nurse at a large West Coast hospital: "I was on duty in coronary care when wild alterations on a patient's EKG indicated possible heart failure. I put in a call for any available doctor to come immediately, and meanwhile I suctioned mucus out of the patient's mouth. Minutes later, a young pediatrician came running toward me. He looked at me dumbly, as if to say, 'What shall I do?'

"I said, 'Fifty milligrams of Xylocaine have proved effective in the past.'

"Then, with a note of authority the doctor ordered, 'Give him fifty milligrams of Xylocaine immediately.'

" 'Thank you, doctor,' I replied."

This form of oblique communication rates a high score for the nurse, and is likely to gain her a reputation for being "damn good." If she refuses to play the game and becomes too assertive, she is punished, labeled a bitch, and considered to be suffering from severe penis envy. She'll be given lots of paperwork and menial chores.

So in addition to lousy hours, mediocre pay, and low status, the nurse must grapple with feelings of powerlessness. Frustration ultimately leads to passivity and the result is that nurses won't report a doctor's error for fear of getting in trouble themselves.

With a changing consciousness and the crisis in health services, new questions are arising: Can the nurse who takes initiative and makes her own decisions survive? Will doctors accept a health-care partnership with nurses? How can society's new needs be met with old training methods? And for the nurse herself, what about the future.

The prognosis looks promising, despite the fact that nurses who are trying to professionalize and adopt "expanded roles" are encountering frustrating obstacles.

The term "expanded role" refers to the nurse's potential for performing functions which have not traditionally been considered within her domain. For instance, a pediatric nurse practitioner can handle preventive care and checkups for the well child, in addition to treating routine and simple illnesses—using the physician only as a backup for serious illness and consultation. The nurse takes over duties ordinarily attended to by the pediatrician, who in turn is freed to spend more time on serious medical problems.

There are also opportunities for a nurse to expand in a general direction by becoming an independent practitioner. The independent nurse practitioner can hang out a shingle, maintain her own or shared offices, see clients, make house calls, and refer cases to a physician when she feels it is necessary. One of the first independent nurses in the country, Lucille Kinlein of San Francisco points out, "No longer is the patient going to be looked on as the concern solely of the physician. This is not right and not necessary. . . I see myself as an extension of the client, *not* of the physician. I am my clients' champion." Kinlein's clients receive treatment for $5 in her office, $10 on a house call. "Health care shouldn't cost an arm and a leg," she contends.

Midwifery is making a triumphant comeback in this country now that laws against it have relaxed. R.N.'s who have taken additional training and have qualified as Certified Nurse-Midwives deliver babies and care for patients before and after birth. "It allows you a continuity and control of the patient that nursing never did," says Judy Carlson, a practicing New York midwife. "Now I can stop a doctor from sedating a woman who wants natural childbirth. As a nurse, I couldn't prevent it." The controversy among the 1,200 or so midwives in this country today is whether to align themselves with the nursing professions, which represents their roots, or with the medical profession, which represents new power and prestige.

The full elasticity of the nurse's role is shown in rural areas where nursing projects, often federally funded, are the only health care available to the poor and disadvantaged. The oldest and probably best example of this kind of daring health care is the Frontier Nursing Service (FNS), founded in 1925. Until recently, horses provided the main transportation for the nurses servicing people who live over the mountains, across the creeks, and through the backwoods of several Kentucky counties. Forty-one nurses, four physicians, and a pharmacist treated over 22,000 patients last year. "We operate under the assumption that nurses are safe practitioners to start out with, and that they will ask if they don't know something," says an FNS staff member. "Nurses know much more than people give them credit for." More important, nurses know enough to recognize when something is beyond their competence.

In 1971, the Department of Health, Education, and Welfare issued a report citing the need for nurses to extend the scope and range of their practice. This year, Nixon's proposed budget cuts all but erase the federally funded training programs necessary for fulfilling HEW's assessment of the nurses' role.

The training programs available vary vastly from state to state in style, length, and title. They are a source of controversy and confusion within the ANA. Many nurses feel the "extended role" is a total non sequitur. "Although today's experts in cardiac and renal surgery bear little resemblance to their historical antecedents—barbers and bloodletters—no one refers to our eminent medical colleagues as 'extended physicians,' nor to their role as 'expanded,' " notes the head of the New York State Nurses Association.

The hospital system has exploited the nursing profession, used its cheap productivity, and ignored its cravings for dignity and respect. And because of insecurity, lack of money, and lack of political power, the profession has cooperated.

But recently the American Medical Association's attempts to create a new job category called the "physician's assistant" (P.A.) has struck many nurses as the final straw.

With fewer than 400 P.A.'s in the entire country, it may seem outrageous that the P.A. issue transforms mild-mannered Dr. Jekylls into Mr. Hydes. Yet this new health-care category, already the subject of a soapsuds TV series, has become a symbolic battleground for the great war between the AMA and the ANA. It began in 1970 when the AMA proposed that "with modest additional training 100,000 nurses could become associated with physicians in such a way as to expand the physician's ability to serve his patients." The nursing organization immediately rejected the idea of the P.A., and continued to demand recognition as members of their own profession (not assistants to the medical profession), and contended that if expanded nursing roles had been recognized sooner, there'd be no need for the P.A.

One of the most disturbing aspects of the new concept is that P.A.'s, most of whom are men at present, have less education and less legal responsibility than the general staff R.N., yet they earn from $200 to $1,200 per year more than the nurse. The P.A. category is designed to be a perfect slot for ex-military corpsmen which the Vietnam War has turned out at the rate of 6,000 a year. And it enables men to join the health-care field without bearing the so-called stigma of the title "nurse."

As the boundaries between nursing and medicine become more and more vague (due to the efforts of nurses, not doctors), the medical profession views the P.A. issue as its last chance at maintaining male control and superiority. In New York two years ago, medical lobbyists managed to get Governor Rockefeller's signature on a law authorizing P.A.'s—at the same time as he rejected the Nurse Practice Act, the ANA's bid to expand its legal scope of practice. Once the P.A. law was passed, and the medical profession had successfully insulated itself against the threatening inroads of nursing practice, state medical and hospital societies slackened their opposition to the Nurse Practice Act. Rockefeller signed that act into law the following year after the P.A. act rendered it toothless and nonthreatening.

While the war over the P.A. issue still rages, a joint committee made up of representatives of the ANA and the AMA is attempting to negotiate a cease-fire. Nevertheless, action continues on other fronts.

The common lament is, "Why have we put up with these conditions for so long?" Calls to action are rarely implemented, and a moving spirit is lacking. The ANA represents only one quarter of the practicing R.N.'s in the country and therefore lacks the power to be pervasive and representative. It has, to date, managed only to inch its way from the status quo.

According to Virginia Cleland, activist and nursing professor at Wayne State University, "We see directors of nursing fighting collective bargaining, written contracts, grievance procedures, et cetera, most often at the request of male administrators. These so-called leaders have risked the lives of patients rather than take forceful public stands to insist on the closing of improperly staffed areas."

An assistant director of nursing admitted, "We know it's our fault for being so meek all these years, but now that many of us are ripe for change, we don't know how to accomplish it, who to look to for leadership, how to organize ourselves. We're like children learning to tie our shoelaces by ourselves for the first time."

Ironically, some nurses are looking for leadership from the men now joining the ranks. But most nurses resent the fact that male nurses, who comprise only 2 percent of the profession, tend to receive faster promotions and salary raises. They frequently end up in leadership positions in their local and state organizations simply because they are not putting up with inequities the way the women have. Both sexes have a way to go before unanimity of interest unites them in the politics of change.

Nurses are going to have to change laws as well as their consciousnesses. Nurses are licensed by the state, ostensibly for the protection of the patient. Now, however, the AMA is pushing for licenses to be issued by institutions, rather than the state. With this eventuality nurses would find themselves completely at the mercy of their male-run institutions with almost no recourse or mobility.

In another area, the ANA filed charges against the nation's largest university pension underwriter for discrimination on the basis of sex. The complaints, filed with the Equal Employment Opportunity Commission by three nursing professors, allege that the Teachers Insurance and Annuity Association "provides larger monthly payments to a male member than to a female member upon retirement at the same age, even though each has made equal contributions for an equal number of years."

Just as women outnumber the male population, so nurses hold a majority among health workers. By uniting, they can wield tremendous power. But first, they must believe that their cause as nurses is an important one.

## Prescription For Action

- Start rap groups where you work. Discuss feminist and nursing issues.
- Present your grievances to management as a group. Be unified about your approach and demands before meeting with the employer. Try to involve as many nurses as possible despite their range of training and experience.
- Join the American Nursing Association. Increase the ANA's clout and get them working for you on the state or national level.
- Join "Nurses for Political Action," a national organization committed to gaining political leverage for the profession. Contact: Marjorie Stanton, % Molloy College, Rockville Centre, Long Island, New York. (516) 678-5000.
- Start a campaign against the image of nurses as presented in the media. Write letters, picket, organize a boycott of newspapers, products, and TV programs.
- Align politically with NOW and/or other local women's organizations so you can increase your base of support and have more women available for actions.
- Start a campaign to raise the consciousnesses of your own doctor or the doctors where you work.
- Know your history. For inspiration we suggest: *Witches, Midwives, and Nurses: A History of Woman Healers,* by Barbara Ehrenreich and Deirdre English. Glass Mountain Pamphlet No. 1 ($1.25 plus 40 cents handling), The Feminist Press, Box 344, Old Westbury, N.Y. 11568.

*—Trucia Kushner*

# The Right to Know, to Decide, to Consent, and to Donate

*Amitai Etzioni*

If you are concerned with one or more of the following questions, you should inform yourself about the new genetics, your chances, your rights, and your opportunities.

— Could you, and should you, be tested to find out if you are carrying in your genes a disease which will send you into a wheelchair later in life? (Researchers have identified more than fifteen hundred illnesses which are partially or completely determined by our genes.)

— If you plan to have a child, do you know the steps you can take *now* to avoid having a retarded child, or a mongoloid (a tragedy which hits one out of every six hundred births in the United States), or a victim of at least a score of other devastating afflictions?

— If some vital organs fail, do you know what will determine whether a replacement can be found? Whether the cash needed will be available? Whether the doctors and nurses and technicians needed will have been trained in the proper techniques?

— As a citizen, should you approve, disregard, or oppose experiments to grow babies in test tubes and to make copies of people?

— Should people with "criminal" genes (XYY) be forbidden to have children?

— And who should make all these decisions? You? Your doctor? The government? A council of wise persons?

These and other questions must be faced in the near future because a new technological revolution is upon us. This revolution, based on developments in both biology and physiology, will do to our genes and brain chemistry what the Industrial Revolution did to our muscle power. Natural processes will become far more subject to human engineering.

**Amitai Etzioni, Ph.D.** is professor of sociology at Columbia University and director of the Center for Policy Research, New York, New York.

The new revolution will expand our capability both to wreak evil and to render good.

To highlight that we are in the initial phase of the age of genetic *engineering*, I refer to a genetic "fix"; we can *now* tamper with our biological inheritance, both fix it where it went wrong and improve it. This article is not primarily a chronicle of new scientific developments; rather, it focuses on your right to know of opportunities and their consequences, your right to be in on the decisions now being thrust upon us.

This somewhat personal article deals chiefly with what I learned and felt when I participated in an international meeting of experts that reviewed these new scientific breakthroughs. It also deals with what I have tried to do about all this and how far I have gotten.

Why a personal account? Because simply to cite what the experts have stated would contribute to the separation of mind and emotion that is the curse of modern civilization. Were I merely to list the number of people who die because kidney machines are not available or because a nationwide tissue-match system has not been organized, I would be giving short shrift to the agony caused by the untrammeled, abused, or unused new technology. Hence, while relevant data are reported, I felt compelled also to attend to the human element behind the figures.

## The Need for Guidance

A good part of what one picks up at a meeting comes not from scientific papers but from the discussions which follow them. In many of these exchanges, I found confirmation for my position that an effective assessment mechanism of the new genetic techniques was badly needed.

One morning over coffee, a participant mentioned that in some countries the death of a donor of organs to be used for transplants is certified only by the surgeons who are to use them and that blatant ethical violations have occurred. Another participant referred to a black market of organs in which body parts suitable for transplants were sold to the highest bidder.

If an international commission were operating, I suggested, it would recommend that the sale of organs be forbidden. Such advice, however, requires additional deliberation, since organs are in very short supply, and paying for them is one way to get more. Maybe "flesh banks" are needed, but two doctors other than the transplant specialist should certify the death of the donor. The commission might also decide that transplant organs should be made available to those who need them on the basis of criteria other than the recipient's ability to pay, such as the general health of the afflicted person, the age, family situation, and other such criteria.

Another area in which the conference reinforced the need for an ethics review board concerned experimentation with humans. Shortly before the conference, newspapers carried reports of experiments conducted on syphilitics in Tuskegee, Alabama. The experiment began in 1932 with about six hundred black men, mostly poor and uneducated, from an area which at the time had the highest syphilis rate in the nation. Though a cure later became available, it was denied to the subjects of this experiment in order to allow the study to complete its run.

In neurophysiology, experiments involving the placement of electrodes into the brain have been made on subjects who have not granted informed consent — they are often being treated for psychosis and epilepsy — and who are not aware of the possibility of subsequent serious brain damage. Despite these often reported abuses, very few countries have statutes limiting experimentation on human subjects.

Another urgent topic was dealt with only briefly during the meeting: the definition of death and concomitant issues. What about dilemmas in the families of patients kept alive by so-called "heroic efforts" once consciousness has been lost and cannot be restored? In most countries, the required judgments are left almost completely to the discretion of the physician. The doctors don't have guidelines emanating from systematic deliberation and based on public consent; therefore, the more progressive doctors lack the support a respected commission could marshal for their new procedures, and public education on the matter is diffuse.

Even less clear are matters which concern the definition of when life begins. Some doctors choose to define life as beginning with conception (a definition which would, of course, outlaw abortions even of mongoloid fetuses); others would wait until the examining pediatrician certified that the born child was alive (allowing them to declare a deformed infant "dead"). The U.S. Supreme Court recently applied the term "viability" in the way some doctors do — that is, as the point at which the fetus can be maintained without a link to the mother's body. However, it did not say whether "viability" includes or excludes the use of machines. With the development of artificial wombs a fetus of any age will become viable once it is removed from the mother.

A commission could do more than define the point at which a fetus acquires the legal and moral status of a human being. It could also help clarify the intricate matters involved in gaining "informed consent" for whatever practitioner or researchers wish to do. But what is the "informed consent" of an unborn child? Should the parents decide for it? British law requires that the court approve *any* experiments on children, not just those performed on fetuses. However, in many countries, children are not protected this way. A thorough and public exploration of these issues is needed. Nothing illustrated this point better than the next session of the conference, by far the most troubling one of all in three turbulent days.

## Two Pediatricians Experiment on Babies

The first speaker was Dr. L. J. Dooren of the department of Pediatrics, University Hospital, Leiden, Netherlands. Dr. Dooren discussed the treatment of infants suffering from severe combined immunodeficiency. These infants are defenseless against attacks by bacteria or viruses. Until four years ago, almost all these infants died within the first year of life.

Dooren reported that some of these infants can now be saved by transplanting bone-marrow cells from a donor. But such a transplantation "will, in practically all cases, lead to lethal graft-versus-host disease unless the donor of the marrow is identical with the patient. If the infant has siblings, then each sibling has one chance in four of having such identity with the patient. Even in such combinations some risk for graft-versus-host disease is present." In short, while one out of four will live, three out of four will die, many from the very therapy administered.

One may say, "Well, they are doomed to die anyway." But there is a difference between a death which cannot be averted and one which is medically induced. Moreover, the death caused by reaction to the transplant is, as Dooren put it, "dehumanizing." When the procedure fails, the infants become violently sick, twisting first in mounting discomfort and nausea and then in excruciating pain as their bodies try to shake off the alien intrusion.

What does it mean, Dr. Dooren asked, for parents to consent to such a transplant? Would they have consented to the transplant if they knew what would be likely to follow?

Aside from the issue of the informed consent of parents for such experiments, questions are raised concerning the consent of the *donors* of the bone marrow. These, mainly siblings of the afflicted infants, are usually children. And as Dooren points out, once the procedure is fully explained to a prospective donor, the donor-child can hardly refuse to participate. The child knows that he or she is the only one who can save the dying sibling. Therefore is the child, once approached, left with a real choice?

But not everyone agrees that people, children included, should be spared either difficult questions or necessary pain.

During the discussion, a theologian pointed out that our culture is intolerant of situations in which people make sacrifices. He observed: "We followed too much the pursuit of happiness and endless life without pain at all. And so we took the dimension of sacrifice out of our life altogether. I do not think it is immoral to ask a member of the patient's family to sacrifice his kidney."

His point was well taken. Surely no one wishes unnecessarily to impose the burdens of such decisions on young children. But it does seem far-fetched to refrain from asking a child to make a life-saving donation that entails only minimal physical risk out of fear that if the child refuses, he or she will feel guilty. However, several psychiatrists considered it "criminal" to place the burden of such a decision on a child, believing that the resulting guilt might cripple a child for life.

We have to formulate some guidelines for these situations. Should a doctor put a child in the position of deciding whether to make sacrifices, even when it is unlikely that the recipient will benefit? And how old must a child be before he or she can be so approached?

The floor was taken next by Dr. Theodore Fliedner, of the University of Ulm in West Germany, who used a different procedure to help children afflicted with basically the same illness. Fliedner's methods avoid the transplant of bone marrow by circulating the infant's blood through a machine, where it is brought into contact with normal blood that contains some of the cells needed to build up immunological defenses. This, it is hypothesized, might stimulate the production of such cells within the afflicted child.

To guard against a reaction to the alien cells introduced through the machine, and to "reduce or eliminate the bacterial flora of his intestinal tract and skin," Fliedner isolates the infant for one year or more.

The results? "In our group, twin boys with a congenital immune-deficiency syndrome have been decontaminated from their microbial flora when they were seven weeks old and maintained in plastic isolation units for more than two point five years . . . there was a gradual development of some immune competence that was encouraging enough to finally introduce a new microbial flora step by step. . . They are now outside the isolator for one year. Although they show intermittent infection, they do quite well."

Questions rushed to mind: Was it sensible to keep a child from birth to age two and a half in a box, to eventually discharge him only to return him to the hospital frequently, to be kept alive for a number of years unknown?

Could a child develop normally in a plastic container? Fliedner reported that psychologists supervised the children to be sure that no ill effects of their confinement occurred

and to work them out if they started to develop. How reliable were those psychological measures that showed "good general development of the children?" Was it wise that these psychologists were consultants to the team rather than part of an independent evaluative procedure?

Fliedner himself did not disregard these issues, and spoke in favor of an autonomous review mechanism. He said experimental therapy needs to be reviewed continuously by appropriate clinical investigation committees, on the basis of accepted ethical rules as — for instance — those laid down in the declaration of the World Medical Association in 1964.

So far, of the 119 children treated by all those involved, at least 87 had died, and only in the case of 12 survivors can one speak of successful treatment and, possibly, the treatment method was advanced. A participant asked both experimenting doctors: "Do you propose to continue with these techniques or not? And if yes, why, since they have such terrible drawbacks?"

Dooren responded: "For the moment my strategy is, if possible, not to treat a new patient before the clinical history of the last patient treated has been fully evaluated and discussed by a team of experts, including experts in the psychological field. . . In this way it has been possible to treat each succeeding patient a little bit better than the former one. With each new patient we have to be very critical concerning the indication for transplantation, and very careful for the patient, the parents, the donor, and the members of the team."

It would be terrible enough to have a child born without immunological defenses. But if the doctors themselves cannot agree on these experimental treatments, how is a parent to choose between them? Do doctors tell their patients that there is a choice? Are Dooren's parents told about Fliedner's work? The issues raised by the kind of information provided to patients, the conditions under which they could provide "informed consent" to experimentalists pointed again to the need for a body such as my pet Health-Ethics Commission, to lead public discussions, education, policy making, and debates on the new procedures that medical services will have to develop to handle these problems.

Another question brought my attention back to the dialogue in the meeting hall. "I may have misunderstood Professor Dooren — indeed I hope I did. But I think I heard him say that blood samples are taken from people, that the samples are typed for the HLA type [the many types of antigens whose development determines the success of tissue transplantation], and that this information is kept on file without these people knowing that they may eventually be asked to donate bone marrow or a kidney for a recipient. Did I hear correctly that this is done without the knowledge of the donor?"

Dooren replied, "These people are not told . . . that the computer may indicate them to be possible donors for bone-marrow transplantation. Is that an answer to your question?"

The questioner stated: "It is an answer to my question, and I regret that I did not misunderstand you. I think this is completely unethical."

I wondered, should the patient's right to know and to consent be treated as an absolute one, even in cases like this?

It seems desirable that when a person's blood is tested it should also be determined whether he or she could serve as a potential organ, blood, or bone-marrow donor. This information should then be kept in a computer, where it would be readily available. Often people die because appropriate donors cannot be found quickly enough.

At the same time to inform someone that he might be called upon one day to donate this or that, would cause many people — most of whom will never be asked — to start worrying about how they might respond if such a request came from strangers or relatives, if it was for a vital organ during life or posthumously, and so forth. On the face of it, the answer seems obvious: wait until an actual need for a decision to donate has arisen before informing them.

The assumption behind this suggestion — to "spare" the masses the burden of reflection, even of anxiety

— is often heard from those opposed to fully informing patients. However, it is a highly paternalistic and patronizing view. People are seen as children to be protected by doctors who know better and who will make the "tough" decisions for them. It seemes to me that people should be told and that the "psychological burden" means, in effect, that people will be given a longer time to think about the issues involved before they may have to make a decision.

Obviously, one cannot say that all doctors should always tell the patients everything. There is a sizeable part of the population — some estimate it to be as high as 25 percent — who are psychologically disoriented even before they are faced with crisis decisions. Studies suggest that when a major anxiety is added to an already critical mass, many "normal" people may suffer a breakdown.

But there is no question in my mind about the direction in which we should move — we should bring people in on as many decisions as possible as soon and as fully as possible. But this should not be done naively, with an untutored reformer's zeal. Opening up to the public, involving the citizen, should be combined with public education on the issues involved as well as institutional and professional reforms.

All this is to illustrate — if it needs more illustration — that at this point most medical decisions are now left almost exclusively to the discretion of the individual practitioner. The reluctance of many doctors to share information with the patient will probably persist until a new consensus is formed in favor of more openness. Without it, those who might be inclined to open up will fear censure from their colleagues as well as damage suits.

As society needs both to protect the doctors from undue pressures so that they will feel free to take reasonable risks and to protect patients from abuse, it might make sense to bar malpractice suits, but to allow persons to file complaints against doctors before local health-ethics commissions. These would be more responsive to complaints because doctors would constitute only a minority position on them, and the commissions could, I suggest, bar a doctor from further practice. Moreover, insurance should be available to patients, rather than to doctors, to support them if they are seriously handicapped by faulty treatment.

Also, many doctors have an authoritarian proclivity and are reluctant to discuss matters in which their patients might want to have a say. If this is to be changed, counterforces will have to be generated to promote a new attitude. Most doctors will not change their bedside manners without considerable encouragement from their more progressive peers, the health authorities, ethical leaders, and, above all, the public.

In recent years there has been grow-ing recognition of the importance of physician-nurse relations to patient care. As technology and specialization has become more complex, however, strains in interprofessional relations have become more apparent. Some have responded to these stresses by role change; others have cried for a return to traditional patterns.

The purpose of the present paper is twofold; to review the literature relevant to these changing roles and relations; and to offer a conceptual framework that may aid in under-standing them.

*"Physicians . . . tend to think of themselves as soloists, disclaiming their need for others. When the doctor does think of the nurse, he tends to view her primarily as his helper, following his orders and carrying out whatever he chooses to delegate."*

# DOCTOR AND NURSE: CHANGING ROLES AND RELATIONS

## *Barbara Bates*

Condensed and reprinted by permission from *The New England Journal of Medicine,* Volume 283, Number 3, pp. 129–134, July 16, 1970.

**Barbara Bates, M.D.** is professor of Medicine, University of Rochester School of Medicine and Dentistry, Rochester, New York.

## MEDICINE AND NURSING — ROLES AND ORIENTATIONS

Medicine and nursing have com-mon goals: the preservation and res-toration of health. Yet their roles in achieving these objectives are not identical. The primary role of medicine comprises diagnosis and treatment — the "cure" process. In contrast, the primary role of nursing lies in the "care" process — expres-sive in nature and consisting of car-ing, helping, comforting and guid-ing.

While emphasizing diagnosis and therapy, medicine has exhorted its members to maintain a broad perception of patient care, to recognize the multiple influences on human health and illness and the needs that these engender. To maintain such a perspective midst the pressures of daily work, however, may be more than the physician can manage. There is evidence to indicate that the doctor limits his perception of patients' problems — organic, psychiatric and social — because of lack of both time and training. Other research has shown that these limitations are greatest in the psychosocial areas. In their study of patient care in a university medical center, Duff and Hollingshead report, "the physician focused his interest on physical disease; he was usually not concerned with personal and social influences in relation to the disease." Other investigators suggest that many physicians are more skilled and comfortable in meeting patients' needs for drugs and for diagnostic or therapeutic technologies than they are in providing a trusting relation and skilled understanding. Despite a variety of educational efforts, both students and practitioners of medicine appear to resist change from this disease-focused point of view.

In contrast with those of medicine, the role definitions and educational programs of nursing might be expected to produce a more psychosocial orientation. Several recent studies have documented this differ-ence between professions, at least in ambulatory-care settings. Two groups of investigators have shown that nurses working in child health clinics place greater emphasis on the family than physicians do. Lewis and Resnik studied pairs of senior medical and senior nursing students participating together in a home-care program. Medical students reported primarily disease-oriented objectives and biologic prognostic factors whereas nursing students described primarily patient-centered objectives and social factors. Thus, the two professions observe the patient from different vantage points and perceive correspondingly different problems.

## THE DOCTOR'S VIEW OF THE NURSE'S ROLE

Unfortunately, the physician does not enjoy a good reputation in his relations with non-physician co-workers. Described as the "last of the autocrats," he tends "to consign the other allied health personnel to a nonprofessional limbo, regarding these persons as working for [him] rather than working for the patient . . . [He] considers these persons as [his] servants rather than as associates or colleagues." He may scarcely consider them at all.

Physicians, then, tend to think of themselves as soloists, disclaiming their need for others. When the doctor does think of the nurse, he tends to view her primarily as his helper, following his orders and carrying out whatever he chooses to delegate.

## THE NURSE'S ACTUAL ROLE IN PATIENT CARE

Observations indicate that his constricted concept of the nurse's role derives not so much from perceptual distortion as from fact. E. L. Brown has described hospital nursing organization as task-oriented rather than patient-oriented. Duff and Hollingshead further document the role of the nurse as physician's assistant and add that the nurse, spending no more time than the doctor in interaction with patients, knew almost nothing about their personal problems. In Schulman's terms, the nurse's "care" has retreated before the "cure" activities that she has accepted from the physician healer.

In summary, when the physician thinks of the nurse, he views her as his technical assistant, and she is just that. Although nursing educators advocate a psychosocial orientation and although nurses may be more person-oriented than their disease-oriented medical colleagues, nursing practitioners have not been notably successful in developing this role.

## ETIOLOGY OF THE CONSTRICTED NURSE ROLE

To understand this constriction of the nurse's role, it may be worthwhile to examine the nature of the physician-nurse relation. There is considerable evidence to indicate

*". . . the nurse's "care" has retreated before the "cure" activities that she has accepted from the physician healer."*

that this relation is characterized by medical authoritarianism on the one hand and nursing's acceptance of dependence or even deference on the other. The development of the full nursing role is thereby limited both by pressures from without and by timidity from within. Reasons for this pattern can be found in medicine, in nursing and in the broader social context of which each is a part.

The physician's role as healer requires not only that he be highly competent but also that he be "decisive, authoritative and assertive." Self-confidence is essential. To recognize a need for others is to acknowledge his limitations. Despite his delegation of tasks, the physician continues to feel a final medical responsibility — ethical and legal — for all that happens to his patient. Levy suggests that this need to control stems partly from feelings of guilt and inadequacy — an occupational hazard of medicine.

Except perhaps for an articulate minority, nurses have not rebelled against the authoritarian physician. Researchers have observed that the average staff nurse in fact accepted a posture of deference toward the physician and was little troubled by this relation.

Reasons for such behavior can be found in nursing traditions that have emphasized obedience and granted few rewards for innovation. Other sociocultural factors contribute. Physicians are usually men, most nurses are women, and the pattern of male dominance prevails. Doctors are usually older, tend to come from a higher socioeconomic class, have a stronger base of knowledge, and have been accorded greater rewards and higher prestige by society.

Factors outside the nature of the interprofessional relation also contribute to the constriction of the nurse's role. The typical medical curriculum has provided the student with little knowledge of the contributions of his colleagues in other disciplines. There may be no formal contact with nurses whatever.

E. L. Brown points out that the ward-based pattern of nursing organization prevents the development of a person orientation. Inadequate education and a relative lack of nursing theory may further contribute to the absence of a more fully developed nursing role. Moreover, the staff nurse may seek to acquire delegated technics as a route to professional prestige.

## PATIENT CARE TODAY

Shaped by all these forces, patient care, today, places its major emphasis on the diagnosis and treatment of disease. The nurse, helping the physician toward this clearly important goal, concentrates her forces on the tasks required. Although she provides physical care to the hospitalized patient, her full potential in guiding, helping and comforting the patient go largely unrealized. Many of the patient's psychosocial needs persist, unidentified and unmet.

## NEW APPROACHES

Stimulated by the recognition that this pattern of patient care is inadequate, leaders within both professions are developing new approaches and roles.

### The Clinical Specialist

One of these is the clinical nurse specialist or nurse clinician. Emphasizing skilled nursing practice, knowledge in depth and recognition of the full spectrum of patient needs, this concept provides substance to the hitherto shadowy nursing role.

Conceptually, the clinical specialist has been considered responsible for the total nursing care of the patient, not simply the delegated tasks of one shift. She may have the freedom to plan her own hours, on the basis of her judgment of patient needs rather than on the exigencies of technical schedules. Little's experience suggests that this role cannot be implemented unless the nurse is explicitly freed from these tasks. Despite the opportunity to effect other kinds of organizational changes, this investigator found it necessary to provide two kinds of nurses to give full patient care — the clinical specialist together with a technically oriented staff nurse.

## The Expanded Role of the Nurse

While the nursing profession has been exploring the clinical specialist's role in a variety of settings, teams of doctors and nurses have tried a second approach, the expanded role of the nurse. Developed primarily in the field of ambulatory care, this role enables the nurse to take on certain responsibilities usually restricted to the physician. With advanced training and experience—for example, in physical examination—this nurse monitors the patient's condition, manages relatively uncomplicated problems, institutes preventive measures and provides emotional support and guidance. She sees patients independently, referring them back to the doctor as indicated. Although she assumes a portion of the physician's traditional role, the concurrent maintenance of her own role is emphasized.

Lewis et al. described a study in which patients were cared for in nurse clinics, amalgamating an expanded nurse role with physician participation. When compared with patients receiving traditional medical-clinic care, their nurse-clinic patients showed less disability, fewer symptoms, fewer broken appointments, fewer criticisms of their care and de-

*"So far as . . . [the nurse's] role is overlapping with medicine, rather than comprising a portion of it, the doctor-nurse team should be able to identify and meet a wider spectrum of patient needs."*

creased use of other medical resources.

Despite such successes, the concept of the expanded role has set off ripples of apprehension within nursing, lest the role be consumed by medicine and deteriorate into an expanded set of delegated tasks. The primarily technical functions of some nurses employed in special clinical and research projects initiated by medicine give just grounds for these fears.

## The Physician's Assistant

A third approach to improving care is the development of a physician's assistant. Medicine is recognizing that many of its activities do not require the full depth of its knowledge. Recognizing at the same time that nurses may not be willing to take on these activities, it is exploring the potentials of an assistant in its own image.

By providing help with less complex medical tasks, this assistant enables the doctor to concentrate his efforts on more difficult problems. Both nursing and medicine may anticipate further problems in interprofessional relations as a physician's assistant is added to an already complicated organization involving doctor, nurse, practical nurse and nursing aide.

## CONCLUDING REMARKS

All these attempts to improve the patterns of patient care are new. Information now available, however, suggests a number of tentative conclusions.

The role of the physician's assistant is still unfamiliar to most medical practitioners, but several factors enhance its chances of acceptance. The points of view and goals of physician and helper are those of a single profession. The assistant's functions are clearly delegated by the doctor and tend to be technicized. Both conditions facilitate the transfer of functions from physician to paramedical personnel and are compatible with medicine's directive pattern of leadership. It seems probable that physician assistants will make their major contributions in the more technical areas of medical practice. There is little evidence that they will move importantly into the psychosocial aspects of patient care or into the helping, comforting and guiding role of the nurse.

In contrast, the nurse in an expanded or specialist role should be equipped to make a broader contribution to patient care. So far as her role is overlapping with medicine, rather than comprising a portion of it, the doctor-nurse team should be able to identify and meet a wider spectrum of patient needs. This pattern of care may be most appropriate to patients with complex or long-term problems. Implementation, however, may meet several obstacles. The nurse's role is more comprehensive than that of the physician's assistant and involves professional responsibility and judgment within her own field. Although a pattern of medical leadership that facilitates communication and involves the nurse in decision making should be more effective in this kind of interprofessional team, it is less characteristic of physician behavior than the directive approach.

Finally, the technology of health care is making enormous demands upon medicine and, through medicine, upon nursing. Despite their complexity, technical aspects of patient care are often more manageable than the psychosocial and interpersonal. They may also be more remunerative, more exciting and less personally disturbing. Whether, amid these pressures and lures, nursing can acquire sufficient knowledge and strength to develop and maintain its own role is a question for the future. Whether medicine can learn to work more effectively with nursing is an equally important issue. The search for answers to these questions will impinge on sensitive areas within both professions, and decisions should be based upon experimentation, reasoned judgment and joint planning.

Reprinted with permission
from *The Journal of Nursing Administration*
November-December 1973

# EXPANDED ROLES FOR PROFESSIONAL NURSES

### by Nathan Hershey

The term *physician extender* is being used increasingly to describe both physician's assistants and professional nurses serving in expanded roles. One of the areas of discussion, if not of conflict, regarding health services today is in regard to the drawing of distinctions between the activities and responsibilities of physician's assistants and of nurses in expanded roles. There

**Nathan Hershey, LL.B.**, is profesor of health law, Graduate School of Public Health, University of Pittsburgh. He is a member of the District of Columbia and New York Bars, the Institute of Medicine, National Academy of Sciences, and has served on committees of the American Hospital Association, the Hospital Association of Pennsylvania, and other health organizations.

Recent legislation recognizes two expanded-role concepts for nurses. One concept involves greater independence to pursue professional nursing; the other concerns provision of medical as well as nursing services by nurses. Legislation fostering the latter concept may serve to increase the availability and improve the delivery of medical services.

are some professionals in these fields who believe that the two kinds of practitioners should be looked at separately and that the differences between them should be emphasized[1]. Others believe that the roles of the physician's assistant and the professional nurse are similar in many respects and that stressing the differences between these health practitioners creates difficulties without attendant benefits[2].

Emotions run high concerning issues related to physician's assistants and nurses in expanded roles. The purpose of this article is to clarify some of the relevant issues and establish the appropriate limits, from the public's point of view, on the use of legislation to impose the views of any segment of the health field regarding the issues related to physician extenders.

The history and rationale of the development of the physician's assistant as a new type of health care practitioner has been reviewed in print frequently. Quite simply, the physician's assistant is to provide health services including (based on the education and experience of the individual physician's assistant) some elements of medical care ordinarily provided by physicians, under the supervision and at the direction of a physician. In no sense is the physician's assistant to be considered an independent health practitioner. Rather, the physician's assistant would always serve as an employee of a physician or an institution engaged in providing health and medical services. From the outset the rationale for preparing physician's assistants has been to provide personnel who, having received substantial amounts of training in medical activities, could help to expand the volume of medical services offered by physicians, especially in underserved areas.

The question has been raised as to whether it was necessary to create the occupational or professional category of physician's assistant, separate and apart from professional nursing. The view has been expressed that the physician's assistant category was necessary to provide a career opportunity for men, particularly veterans with military medical experience, who would not want to become professional nurses, but who desired responsible positions in the provision of health and medical services[3].

The question is academic now, because the category of physician's assistant exists and has received legislative recognition in a considerable number of states. Also, a substantial number of educational programs have been established to prepare men and women for careers as physician's assistants, and, while these programs are far from uniform, their basic thrust is clearly to provide health personnel in a role immediately subordinate to physicians.

The idea of expanded roles for professional nurses is not new. The scope of practice of the professional nurse has been enlarged with the passage of time. This process of change can be noted in the joint statements of medical and nursing organizations and opinions of state attorneys general regarding what nurses may do, the variety of educational programs for nurses, and the responsibilities imposed upon nurses in hospitals and other institutions to recognize and to report below-standard medical care endangering patient safety.

Two different concepts of the expanded role of the nurse are becoming evident from positions taken by nursing organizations and from legislative developments. One expansion concept is based upon the nurse as a practitioner who is to be granted greater independence to pursue a discipline called *professional nursing*. Implicit in this concept is the attempt to create for the professional nurse a role comparable to that of the physician, an independent practitioner. Carried to its extreme, the professional nurse would serve individual patients in the same fashion the attending physician serves his private patients, with the nurse functioning in an entrepreneurial capacity. The nurse would enter into contractual relationships with patients for the planning of their nursing care and for general direction and some supervision of the institutional employees, including professional nurses and other nursing service personnel who would render the nursing care on a regular basis. The nurse in the entrepreneurial capacity might maintain an office, see patients there, and charge fees for such services as she renders in dealing with the social, physiological, and psychological needs that affect the health status of patients. In this conception of professional nursing as a parallel to medicine and a clearly separate profession, much reliance is placed on advanced academic study. Not all currently practicing professional nurses would be considered qualified, or even candidates, for such practice according to the advocates of this expanded role concept.

The most serious problem the author has encountered regarding the scope of nursing practice has been in finding legal bases for allowing nurses with suitable qualifications to render services that include in part the making of judgments which appear, to some extent, to involve medical diagnosis, and the selection of therapeutic measures without contemporaneous orders from a physician. The problem is most frequently manifested in two settings: In the provision of primary care at a satellite facility or remote location, and in the furnishing of very specialized care on units in hospitals where decisions must be made quickly and therapeutic measures instituted promptly because of the acute condition of the patients.

A recent legislative development in Idaho, evidently directed at providing a basis for nurses to accept medical responsibilities, reveals an expanded role of the nurse fundamentally different from the one described earlier. An amendment to the Idaho nursing practice act removes the blanket prohibitions of "acts of medical diagnosis or prescription of medical therapeutic or corrective measures" by professional nurses[4]. The amendment permits the state boards of nursing and medicine to jointly promulgate rules and regulations under which professional nurses may carry out such functions. Rules and regulations in accordance with the legislation have been issued, along with examples of what nurses may undertake to do consistent with them. Qualified professional nurses can be employed, consistent with these rules and regulations, to provide some primary medical care in the State of Idaho. While such care technically might be viewed still as medical care, to the extent it is rendered by professional nurses, one can argue that it is "nursing care" also.

Legislative change specifically dealing with expanded roles for nurses has also taken place in the State of New Hampshire[5]. The nursing practice act was amended to permit acts by professional nurses "under emergency or other special conditions . . . as are recognized by the medical and nursing professions as proper to be performed by a professional nurse under such conditions, even though such acts might otherwise be considered diagnosis and prescription." This legislative language appears to be closer in concept to the Idaho nursing practice act amendment than to the new definition in the New York law, because it does not emphasize the distinctions between professional nursing and medicine and it allows nurses to engage in diagnosis and prescription under "emergency or other special conditions." However, some guidance from the state boards would seem to be necessary to delineate the scope of "special conditions."

At this point it is necessary to return to consideration of the term *physician extender* and to determine how it relates to the differing conceptions of the nurse in the expanded role. The concept of the professional nurse practicing a discipline distinct and apart from medicine is not consistent with the term physician extender for the very reason that while a nurse engaged in such nursing practice may be increasing the provision of service to patients, that nurse is not increasing the supply or volume of medical services. On the other hand, nurse practitioners engaged in primary care in clinics and health centers and in satellite facilities of large institutions and who perform medical services are clearly encompassed by the physician extender. In many respects the latter type of nurse in an expanded role is very similar to the physician's assistant. To the extent that the nurse practitioner provides services generally recognized as medical in nature, in addition to traditional nursing services, the nurse must do so subject to some degree of medical supervision and direction, although the physician may be at a different location at the time services are provided. In a

sense, the nurse in the expanded role who functions in this context is subordinate to the responsible medical practitioner, as is the physician's assistant. While the nurse practitioner may undertake many functions that are clearly recognized as nursing, and with regard to them make judgments and apply techniques in a basically independent fashion, the nurse, nevertheless, is providing care to a patient for whom a physician has at that time the overriding responsibility for medical care. Thus, this nurse provides both nursing services and medical services, as distinct from nurses who may, according to the concept embodied in the amended New York nursing practice act, provide only nursing care, which includes, of course, executing specific medical orders.

Few states have changed their legislation as yet to authorize specifically the provision of medical services by professional nurses serving in an expanded role, although, as already described, this has been done in Idaho, New Hampshire, Arizona, and Washington. A greater number of states have established by legislation authority for physician's assistants to engage in the provision of medical services.

This state of affairs raises a serious question for the nursing profession. From the nursing literature it is evident that some nurses believe that professional nurses should reject engaging in the provision of medical services, particularly the tasks and responsibilities that physicians are becoming increasingly willing to delegate to nonphysicians. Instead, they urge nurses to expand their functions within a definition of professional nursing as a discipline clearly distinct and apart from medicine. Those who support this view are certainly entitled to their position, and they may well be pointing toward a type of professional development that will give great satisfaction to nurses who choose to go that route in their careers. However, there are many indications that considerable numbers of practicing nurses desire to increase clinical responsibilities in areas that are generally regarded as medical services.

Opportunities for these nurses to become physician extenders should be fostered both by nursing organizations and by others — physicians, health planners, hospital executives — concerned with increasing the availability of medical services. This recommendation is with full recognition that when professional nurses seek to function as physician extenders, responsibility for their approval as qualified to so function must rest, at least in part, with persons able to determine whether such nurses can provide medical services at an acceptable level. And physician participation in educational programs for nurses seeking this type of expanded role and in approval processes would indicate to the public that the nurses possess the necessary qualifications. With regard to the approval process, this is essentially the system that has been established in Idaho for nurses serving in expanded roles that encompass important elements of medical service.

Meriting consideration in this regard is whether, and to what extent, the approval process for a professional nurse in the expanded role, whose scope of practice will include medical services, might best be accommodated at this time through physician's assistant legislation. Assuming that objective standards are to be utilized by the boards or agencies given responsibility for determining the suitability of individuals for recognition as physician's assistant, there would appear no great difficulty in using the same standards to provide equivalent recognition for qualified professional nurses serving as physician extenders.

Physician's assistant legislation clearly provides that medical services are rendered under physician supervision by those who gain approval according to such legislation. Of course, one might anticipate that some segments of organized nursing would reject the notion that nurses obtain legal authority to engage in certain aspects of patient care through a physician-dominated approval mechanism. Nevertheless, as long as the agencies or boards are willing to do so, and there are applicants seeking such recognition, there is no reason why, at least from the public's point of view, impediments should be imposed by nurses or by any other group to the use of physician's assistant legislation to provide recognition for such qualified nurses.

The author's experience in dealing with questions of scope of practice for nurses, and the accommodation of both physician's assistants and nurses in expanded roles within the health service system, strongly suggests that many problems raised with regard to physician extenders are more apparent than real. Unfortunately, many of the questions that arise are viewed, not from the public's interest broadly conceived, but rather from the point of view of professional and educational organizations seeking to maintain and to reinforce their power or control over activities and people. There is nothing inherently wrong in organizations and institutions seeking to protect and enhance their positions relative to others. We accept that as part of the interplay within our society. However, assertions by vested interests that they are serving the public rather than seeking to achieve their own particular goals, need to be studied carefully, not taken at face value. Furthermore, it is a misuse of the legislative and administrative processes to block the enactment of worthwhile legislation or impede the implementation of such legislation. Physicians who personally do not wish to provide service to their patients through physician extenders are not forced to do so in states in which physician's assistant legislation exists or the nursing practice act permits nurses to perform in expanded roles that encompass medical services. The opportunity for nurses to receive approval to provide medical services as part of an expanded role in no way limits the freedom of nurses who do not desire to engage in such activity from eschewing that route of career development.

In the final analysis, limitations on career opportunities, whether for physician extenders or other types of health personnel or, for that matter, anyone in society, should not be imposed because of parochial interests. These interests will always be with us, but they should be recognized for what they are, rather than what they proclaim themselves to be.

## REFERENCES

1. See Rogers, M.E. Nursing: To be or not to be? *Nurs. Outlook* 20:42-46, 1972; Schorr, T. M. An important distinction. *Am. J. Nurs.* 72:1581, 1972; American Nurses Association, *Statement re Physician's Assistants,* December 17, 1971; New York State Nurses Association, *Statement on the Physician's Associate and Specialist's Assistant,* January 31, 1972.

2. See Lambertson, E.C. The role of nurse practitioners and their relationship to the emerging physician's assistant concept, *Physicians Associate,* October, 1972, pp. 132-135.

3. See *New Members of the Physician's Health Team: Physician's Assistants,* Report of the Ad Hoc Panel on New Members of the Physician's Health Team of the Board on Medicine of the National Academy of Sciences, 1970, p. 2. Note that the early Medex training programs enrolled former military medical personnel exclusively.

4. Idaho Code Ann. §54-1413 (Supp. 1972).

5. N.H. Rev. Stat. Ann. §362-A:2 (Supp. 1972).

# ORIGINAL SOURCES OF ARTICLES

For the convenience of readers who wish to refer to the unabridged versions of articles appearing in this book, we are happy to provide the addresses of the publications in which the articles originally appeared.

Adult Leadership
Adult Education Association of the U.S.A.
810-18th Street, N.W.
Washington, D.C. 20006

American Vocational Journal
American Vocational Association, Inc.
1510 N. Street, N.W.
Washington, D.C. 20005

Annals of Internal Medicine
American College of Physicians
4200 Pine Street
Philadelphia, PA 19104

AORN Journal
Association of Operating Room Nurses
8085 East Prentice Avenue
Englewood, CO 80110

Atlantic Monthly
Atlantic Monthly Company
8 Arlington Street
Boston, MA 02116

Doubleday and Company, Inc.
277 Park Ave.
New York, NY 10017

Journal of Health and Social Behavior
American Sociological Association
1001 Connecticut Ave., N.W.
Washington, D.C. 20036

Journal of The American Medical Association
535 N. Dearborn Street
Chicago, IL 60610

Journal of The New York State Nurses Association
Executive Park East
Stuyvesant Plaza
Albany, NY 12203

Journal of Nursing Administration
12 Lakeside Park
Wakefield, MA 01880

Journal of Nursing Education
Charles B. Slack, Inc.
6900 Grove Rd.
Thorofare, NJ 08086

Journal of Obstetric Gynecologic and Neonatal Nursing
Harper and Row Publishers, Inc.
2350 Virginia Ave.
Hagerstown, MD 21740

MacMillan Publishing Co., Inc.
866 Third Ave.
New York, NY 10022

Ms. Magazine
Ms. Magazine Corporation
370 Lexington Ave.
New York, NY 10017

New England Journal of Medicine
10 Shattuck Street
Boston, MA 02115

Nursing Forum
Nursing Publications, Inc.
P.O. Box 218
Hillsdale, NJ    07642

Nursing '74
430 Benjamin Fox Pavilion
Jenkintown, PA  19046

PRISM
American Medical Association
535 North Dearborn
Chicago, IL  60610

Saturday Review, Inc.
380 Madison Avenue
New York, NY    10017

Science News
Science Service, Inc.
1719 N Street, N.W.
Washington, D.C.    20036

The Sciences
New York Academy of Sciences
2 East 63rd Street
New York, NY    10021

Social Work
National Association of Social Workers
2 Park Ave.
New York, NY    10016